JUICING FOR BEGINNERS:

1000 Days of Natural and Tasty Juicing Recipes to Detox Your Organism, Boost Your Energy, Fight Disease and Lose Weight

Copyright © 2022
Sarah Roslin

TABLE OF CONTENTS

1 Introduction

The health of each organ and cell in the human body is determined by the food we eat. Food can either help us or destroy us. Juicing is the most effective approach to receiving all of the nutrients and vitamins we require on a daily basis to stay healthy.

We're talking about freshly pressed organic vegetable and fruit juice, not store-bought bottled or processed variants. Fresh, plant-based foods provide us with nutritional benefits that processed foods do not. Processed foods are high in calories and lacking in nutrients. Fresh juice is not pasteurized, as is required by the FDA, unlike prepackaged or prepared juices. Even though pasteurization is supposed to protect, the heating procedure can destroy much of the nutritious value.

Both juicing and blending entail transforming fruits and vegetables into a drinking liquid, but that is about the extent of their resemblance.

Juicing is the product r of extracting liquid from fruits and vegetables while removing the particles to make juice. The skin, seeds, and pulp are removed during the extraction process and spit out at the back of the juicing machine.

Blending involves whole fruits or vegetables (or whatever other components you desire) to make them smooth. There is no extraction of the peel, seeds, or pulp (unless you remove them ahead of time). As a result, everything that enters the mixer ends up in your drink.

The reasoning is straightforward: whole, living foods give the optimum nutrition for living beings. Fresh juice is of the highest quality, has immediate bioavailability, and provides immediate and practical benefits. The best approach to receiving all of the nutrients we need each day is to drink the juice of a variety of raw vegetables and fruits.

Fresh juices are the most efficient way to acquire all of the nutritional values of fruits and vegetables. Juicing extracts essential minerals and vitamins. Digestive enzymes, which are primarily found in raw foods, play a variety of essential roles in our health, including turning food into body tissue and energy. One of the finest ways to get active enzymes is to drink fresh juices. Enzymes are also necessary for metabolism. As a result, drinking fresh juices can help you burn more calories. More energy and calories are expended when your metabolic rate is higher. According to the Dietary Guidelines for Americans, 5–13 servings of mixed fruits and vegetables are required each day. This is the equivalent of 61/2–8 cups of fruits and vegetables every day.

One of the significant benefits of juicing is that you can obtain more nutrients in fewer servings than you could with blending. In addition, because you aren't eating whole fruit or vegetable, juices are usually lower in calories. Juicing is a great method to add nutritious snacks or drinks to your diet in this way.

Juicing helps your body absorb nutrients by breaking down fruits and vegetables. Because there is nothing for your digestive system to break down, your body may swiftly obtain energy or calories from juice. When you're fighting an illness, juicing can help your immune system. In fact, because of the benefits and healing effects of juicing, many people who are through chemotherapy turn to it.

Juicing is life-changing, providing more energy, better sleep, stronger immune systems, brighter complexion, and a more youthful appearance. It's even assisting in the recovery of human bodies from a variety of ailments. Juicing on a regular basis is an excellent option for individuals who wish to improve the balance of their diets with a minimal commitment of time, money, and effort. You may add juicing into your daily routine without having to give up your favorite foods or spend countless hours in the kitchen. It takes absolutely no time to prepare and is much faster and easier.

2 Tips for storing juice

1. You can store the juices in the refrigerator for 24 to 48 hours and up to 72 hours at the most.
2. Keep your juices in airtight glass containers.
3. After you've made your juices store them right away.
4. Fill your juice container to the top as much as possible to prevent oxygen exposure.
5. Make Sure You Freeze The Juice Properly!
6. The Container Should Be Vacuum-Sealed
7. Add a piece of citrus to your juice, like lemon, or lime, to reduce nutrient loss by boosting vitamin C, citric acid, and other antioxidants.
8. When traveling, keep your juices in a cold and dark place; it is preferred to use a cooler bag with ice to avoid nutrient loss.
9. If you freeze your juice, it will keep for 12 to 16 months.

3 Washing product

1. Before and after preparing fruits or vegetables, wash your hands for 15-20 seconds in warm water with hand wash or soap.
2. Stir add 1 1/3 cup vinegar and 1 tablespoon salt until they are completely dissolved.
3. Fruits and vegetables should be rinsed and gently rubbed while being placed under running water.
4. Soak thin-skinned fruits/vegetables (such as berries and leafy greens) for 5 minutes and firm-skinned fruits/vegetables (such as apples and squash) for 10 minutes in your vinegar and salt solution, then rinse under running plain water.
5. Scrub hard fruits or vegetables like melons, carrots, sweet potatoes and cucumbers with a clean vegetable brush while washing.
6. Dry fruits and vegetables with a clean kitchen cloth or paper towel to further minimize bacteria.
7. Cutaway damaged or bruised areas of product to prevent bacteria.

4 Fruits, Vegetables, Additives

Fruits	Vegetables
Apple	Carrot
It is a healthy food choice, rich in fiber and vitamin C.	It is high in minerals, vitamins, and antioxidants, also a good source of antioxidants.
Pros:	Pros:
Improve brain health	Vision
Improve gut	Blood pressure and cardiovascular health
Lower cancer risk	Bone health and healing
Lower chronic conditions risk	Cancer
Lower diabetes risk	Diabetes control
Lower heart disease risk	Digestive health
Cons:	Immune function
Blood sugar fluctuations	Cons:

Fruits	Vegetables
Consuming pesticides Digestive issues Gain weight Gastrointestinal distress Pesticide residues	Bloating Constipation Gastrointestinal issues
Orange It is rich in potassium, vitamin C, flavonoids, and fiber. Pros: Boosts immune system Defense against germs Fight anemia Heals wounds Helps in making collagen Improve vision Protects cells Smoother skin Strong immune system Cons: Bloating Can damage bones Cramping Diarrhea Heart attack Heartburn Imbalance blood sugar levels Insomnia Nausea Upset stomach Vomiting	Celery It is a low-fat, low-calorie high in fiber and sodium, loaded with vitamins and minerals with a low glycemic index. Pros: Alkalizing effect Reduces inflammation Supports digestion Cons: Can cause sensitivity to the sun
Pineapple It is packed with nutrients, antioxidants, and other helpful compounds. Pros: Boost metabolism Cleaning the blood Cleaning the organs Help in digestion Nourish nails Nourish skin Nourish your hair Protect against inflammation Provide energy Strong teeth	Lime It is high in vitamin C and antioxidants — both of which may offer health benefits. Pros: Aid iron absorption Improve immunity Prevent kidney stones Promote healthy skin Reduce heart disease risk Cons: Acid reflux Difficulty swallowing Heartburn Nausea

Fruits	Vegetables
Cons: Abdominal pain Diarrhea Heartburn Mouth tenderness Nausea Vomiting	Potential side effects Vomiting
Pear It is a powerhouse packing fiber, vitamins, and beneficial plant compounds. A medium-sized pear contains approximately a hundred calories and is fat-free. Pears are a rich source of dietary fats. Pros: Anti-inflammatory properties heart health booster Help in weight loss Lower diabetes risk Offer anticancer effects Promote gut health Cons: Diarrhea Headache Heartburn Indigestion Liver scarring Nausea Obesity Stomach bloating Vomiting	Ginger It is loaded with antioxidants and compounds. They may help your body fight against chronic diseases. Pros: Alleviates motion sickness Enhances absorption of nutrients Fight heart disease Fight high blood pressure Fight lungs disease Helps fight common respiratory problems Helps with digestion Improves blood flow Minimizes pain and inflammation Prevents cold and flu Promote healthy aging Strengthens immunity Cons: Gas Heartburn. Mouth irritation Upset stomach
Berries They contains several vitamins and minerals, especially vitamin C, and are primarily made up of carbs and fiber. Pros: Boost immunity Fight cavities Fight heart disease Healthy bones Lower cholesterol Manage diabetes Promote heart health Protect against cancer Reduce blood pressure	Cucumber It contains low calories but is high in many essential vitamins and minerals. Pros: Aid in Weight Loss. Lower Blood Sugar Promote Regularity Promotes Hydration Cons: Burping Flatulence Growling Indigestion problems

Fruits	Vegetables
Stomach ulcers Treat urinary tract infections Cons: Bloating Blood sugar spikes, excessive consumption Cause a rash Constipation Diarrhea Gas Headaches Nausea Reflux Risk of kidney stones in predisposed individuals Upset stomach Vomiting	
Blood orange It is full of anthocyanin, vitamin c, and other nutritious. Pros: Anti-cancer properties Anti-inflammatory Decreasing the chance that cells will become cancerous. Reduce damage from free radicals Strong immune system Cons: Can damage blood sugar levels Can damage bones Heartburn Regurgitation	Spinach It is a rich source of zeaxanthin and carotenoids that can flush out the free radicals from your body. Pros: Aids in bone Health Aids in Weight Loss Has Anti-inflammatory Properties Improve eye health Keeps Your Body Relaxed Prevent cancer Reduce blood pressure levels Reduce oxidative stress Reduces Blood Sugar Reduces Hypertension Cons: Abdominal pain Bloating Cramps Diarrhea Gas Sometimes fever Takes time to get digested
Kiwi Kiwi is rich in nutrients but has no fat. It is not a calorie-rich fruit. Pros: Improve immunity Improve skin health	Lemon It is a excellent source of Vitamin C, which is a vital nutrient in preventing many modern diseases. Pros: Boosting immunity Help in weight loss

Fruits	Vegetables
Support digestive health	Prevent regular consumption
Support heart health	Reduce the risk of heart disease
Cons:	Reduce the risk of stroke
Allergic reactions	Cons:
Asthma	Dental erosion
Hives	Headaches
Mouth irritation	Heartburn
Oral Allergy Syndrome	Migraine
Rashes on the body	
Swelling in the body	
Grapes	Sweet potato
They are loaded with natural sugar and over consumption of foods with rich sugar content.	It is a low-fat contains many beneficial nutrients essential to your health. Particularly rich in vitamins, especially vitamin A, fiber, and antioxidants.
Pros:	
Help protect against cancer	Pros:
Help protect against cardiovascular disease	Enhance Brain Function
Prevent eye problems	Fight Cancer
Cons:	Help improve heart health
Cough	Help regulate blood pressure
Diarrhea	Improve nervous system
Dry mouth	Promote Gut Health
Headache	Provide Healthy Vision
	Cons:
	Accumulates in the liver
	Hypervitaminosis
	Increase the risk of calcium-oxalate
	Kidney stones
Melon	Beetroot
It contains low calories but is high in antioxidants, electrolytes, and water, perfect for summer.	It is highly nutritious and loaded with health-promoting properties.
Pros:	People suffering from stone problems should not include beetroot in their diet. It poses a risk to those having some kind of iron and copper condition.
Antioxidant	
Gut growth	
Healthy blood sugar levels	
Healthy eye function.	Pros:
Improving digestive health	Boost athletic performance
Maintenance of cells in the body	Help alleviate inflammation
Promotes bowel regularity	Improve digestive system
Cons:	Slow the growth of cancer cells
Diarrhea	Support brain health heart
High blood sugar levels	Cons:
	Chills

Fruits	Vegetables
	Fever
	Hives
	Itching
	Skin rash
	Swallowing
	Vocal cords to shrink
Apricot	Kale
Have a fair amount of potassium. And potassium plays an essential role in the proper functioning of the heart.	Provides a vast amount of nutrients for a low amount of calories.
Pros:	Pros:
Anti-inflammation	Aids in cold
Reduce diabetes risk	Blood clotting
Reduce heart disease risk	Bone building
Reduce obesity risk	Boost of antioxidants
Treat inflammatory illnesses	Brain development
Cons:	Chronic disease prevention
Faintness	Improve bones health
Giddiness	Improve eye health
Losing consciousness	Improves Cholesterol Levels
Sweating	Improves Immune System
Vomiting	Reduce cancer risk
	Reduces the risk of glaucoma
	Strong immune system
	Cons:
	Bloating
	Can harm thyroid function
	Causing gas
	Constipation
	Diarrhea.
	Toll on the gastrointestinal system
Peach	Mint leaves
It is an amazing source of antioxidants, and peach peels offer the highest level of anticancer properties.	They are in nutrients and a good source of vitamin A, a fat-soluble vitamin. People with gastroesophageal reflux disease (GERD) should not use mint.
Pros:	Pros:
Healthy eyes	Acne-free skin
Healthy heart	Beat morning sickness
Healthy skin	Beat nausea
Improved allergy symptoms	Boosts immune system
Improved digestion	Help with asthma
Strong immune system	Helps with allergies
Cons:	Improve eye health
Coughing	

Fruits	Vegetables
Mild allergy Skin rash Vomiting	Improve night vision Treat cold Treats stomach woes Cons: Abdominal pain Allergic reactions Dry mouth Heartburn Nausea Trigger asthma
Pomegranate it is loaded with vitamin C, vitamin K, potassium, and several other vital nutrients. Pros: Contains antibacterial properties Provides anti-oxidants Reduce the risk of heart disease Cons: Cause gastric issues High in Sugar Poses a risk to those having high sugar levels	Parsley Many vitamins, minerals, and antioxidants can provide essential health benefits. It is loaded with vitamin K. Pros: Reduce cancer risk Reduce diabetes risk Reduce heart disease risk Reduce stroke risk Cons: Anemia Kidney problems Liver problems Skin allergic
Plum It is loaded with vitamins, minerals, fiber, and antioxidants. Pros: Boost body's production Improve bone health Reduce bone loss Slow down blood sugar spike Cons: Diarrhea Gas Stomach issues	Lettuce It is loaded with vitamin K, which helps strengthen bones. Pros: Hydration Improved Sleep Improved Vision Strengthen bones Cons: Allergic reactions Consumption Diarrhea Stomach cramps Vomiting
Banana It is a great source of carbohydrates and quick energy. Pros:	Serrano pepper Contains a variety of health-boosting compounds and is a good source of vitamin A. Pros:

Fruits	Vegetables
Aid weight loss	Excellent for weight loss
Help you feel fuller	Immune System Booster
Improve insulin sensitivity when unripe	Cons:
Support digestive health	Burning aftertaste
Support heart health	
Cons:	
Bloating	
Cramping	
Gas	
High blood sugar levels	
Nausea	
Softer stools	
Vomiting	
Papaya	Onion
It is a good source of fiber.	It is low in calories but loaded with vitamins and minerals.
Pros:	Pros:
Aiding in digestion	Encourage healthy heart
Improving blood glucose	Improved bone health
Improving wound healing	Lower blood sugar levels
Lowering blood pressure	Lowering blood pressure
Lower heart disease risk	Lowering heart attack risk
Lower cancer risk	Reduced risk of cancer
Lower diabetes risk	Cons:
Lower heart disease risk	Asthma
Cons:	Itchy eyes
Cause allergies	Itchy nose
Cause respiratory disorders	Itchy rash
Harmful for pregnant women	Nasal congestion
Lead to digestive issues	Red eyes
Lower blood sugar significantly	Runny nose
Guava	Bell peppers
It s a source of vitamin C, fiber, and other substances that act as antioxidants.	They are low in calories and are loaded with good nutrition.
Pros:	Pros:
Aid healthy bowel movements	Blood sugar-lowering
Good for diabetes.	Delay age-related memory loss.
Have anti-aging properties.	Reduce the likelihood of anemia.
Helps treat constipation.	Reduce the risk of cataract degeneration.
Improve brain health.	Reduce the risk of macular degeneration.
Improve immune system.	Cons:
Improves heart health.	Diarrhea
Prevent constipation	Stomach pain

Fruits	Vegetables
Reduces the risk of developing cancer. Cons: Prone to cold Prone to cough	Trigger allergies Trigger burning sensation
Sapota It s a wholesome fruit that abounds with all essential nutrients, including dietary fibers, iron, calcium, antioxidants, and vitamins A. Pros: Bolsters Immunity Boost Energy Controls Blood Pressure Healthy Skin Prevents Cancer Promotes Gut Health Stronger Bones Cons: Abdominal Pain Allergic Reactions Digestive Issues Inflammation Itching Not Healthy for Diabetic Patients	**Chives** They provide amazing health benefits as they are rich in plant-based antioxidants and nutrients. Pros: Fight inflammation Help fight cancer Improve heart health Cons: Allergic skin reactions Indigestion Stomach pain
Mango It is rich in fiber. Pros: Healthy plant compounds Immune-boosting Improve digestive health Support eye health Supports heart health Cons: Diarrhea Difficulty in breathing Harmful for diabetes patients Runny nose Sneezing Stomach pain	Hearts of Romaine It is a crispy salad green with high nutritional value. Pros: Helps keep bones High in antioxidants Strong teeth Support the immune system Cons: Increase risk of E. Coli Increase the risk of foodborne illnesses
Passion fruit It has low-calorie properties and high nutrients, fiber, and antioxidants. Pros:	Tomato It contains folate and some essential nutrients such as vitamin B, vitamin C, and lycopene. Pros:

Fruits	Vegetables
Boosts immune system Improve insulin sensitivity Low glycemic index Reduce anxiety Supports heart health Cons: Can cause cyanide poisoning	Anti-inflammatory properties Boost immune system Support brain health Support overall heart health Cons: Acid reflux Heartburn
Cherry It is low in calories and loaded with fiber, vitamins, minerals, nutrients, and other essential ingredients. Pros: Anti-inflammatory compounds Benefits heart health Boost exercise recovery Packed with nutrients Rich in antioxidants Cons: Bloating Cramps Intestinal gas	Jalapeno It is loaded with vitamins C-A and potassium. They also have carotene -- an antioxidant. Pros: Help fight cells damage Cons: Diarrhea Stomach pain Trigger a burning sensation
Watermelon It has high water content and also provides some fiber. Pros: Aid skin health Anticancer effects Contains plant compounds Improve heart health Prevent macular degeneration Reduce inflammation Reduce oxidative stress Relieve muscle soreness Stay hydrated Cons: Cardiovascular Problems Diarrhea Digestive Problems Increase The Risk Of Developing Liver Inflammation Up Glucose Levels	Courgette It contains 0% fat and loaded with water and fiber. It also contains nice amount of vitamins B6, riboflavin, folate, C, and K. Pros: Anti-inflammatory properties Lower risk of heart disease Cons: Digestive issues
Fig	Garlic

Fruits	Vegetables
It is a highly nutritious fruit having fibre, potassium, and antioxidant content. Pros: Promotes digestive health Rich in antioxidants Support bone health Support healthy blood pressure Cons: Allergies Diarrhea Digestive symptoms content	It is widely famous for its ability to fight bacteria, viruses, fungi, and even parasites. Pros: Antibiotic Properties Boost Your Immune System Improve Athletic Performance Prevent Alzheimer's Prevent Cancer Prevent Dementia Reduce Cholesterol Levels Reduce High Blood Pressure Cons: Bad breath Diarrhea Gas Heartburn
Litchis It is loaded with vitamin C, vitamin B2 (riboflavin), potassium, and copper. Pros: Antiviral Property Boost immune system Contains Anti-influenza Activity Controls Blood Pressure Effective against cancer Help in digestion Cons: Cause internal bleeding Fever High sugar content Hormonal imbalance	Bottle ground It is rich iron, vitamins and potassium. Pros: Benefits the heart Helps in digestion Helps in weight loss Prevents premature greying of hair Reduces stress Treating sleeping disorders Cons: Diarrhea Discomfort Feeling of uneasiness Nausea Toxic to body Vomiting
Avocado Avocados are a high-fat food, making them one of the fattiest plant foods. Pros: Aid in Weight Loss Balance Blood Pressure Help in Growth and Development Support Healthy Eyes Support Heart Health Cons: Coronary artery disease	Broccoli It has excellent nutritional values. It is rich in fiber, loaded with vitamin C and has potassium, B6, and vitamin A. Pros: Contains cancer protective Good eye health Good for heart health Support hormonal balance Support immune system Cons:

Fruits	Vegetables
Increase risk of obesity Type 2 diabetes	Bloating Digestive distress Excessive gas Irritable bowel syndrome
Black currant It is loaded with vitamin c, containing at least 85% of human daily recommended value in a single serving. Pros: Ease flu symptoms Help strengthen the immune system Soothe sore throats Cons: Belching Diarrhea Gas Headache	Fennel bulb It is low in calories but rich in nutrients linked to many health benefits. Pros: Collagen synthesis Improve immune health Tissue repair Cons: Chest pain Difficulty breathing Hives. Itchiness Nausea Rash. Swollen skin Tightness of chest/throat Vomiting
	Swiss Chard It is a loaded nutritious leafy vegetable. Only one cup contains over three times the vitamin K needed of human daily nutrition. Pros: Cancer prevention Maintenance of heart Maintenance of kidneys Maintenance of lungs Cons: Can lead to kidney stones
	Cauliflower It is high in fiber and water. Plus. Healthy digestive tract Preventing constipation Support hormonal balance Support immune system Cons: Bloating Flatulence

Fruits	Vegetables
	Radish It is a great source of vitamin C. Pros: Helpful for lowering high blood pressure Lower heart disease risk Cons: Cramps Flatulence Irritate the digestive tract
	Purple Cabbage It has anti-cancer properties due to the presence of glucosinolates and anti-oxidants. Pros: Healthier heart Improved gut function Reduce the risk of certain cancers Reduced inflammation Stronger bones Cons: Diarrhea Hypothyroidism Medication interactions
	Asparagus Rich in Antioxidants, also an excellent source of antioxidants like Vitamin A and Vitamin E. Pros: Healthy pregnancy outcomes Help in weight loss Improved digestion Lower blood pressure Cons: Cause flatulence Gastric upset Stomach cramps
	Peas They are loaded with fiber and antioxidants and have properties that may reduce several diseases risk. Pros: Help reduce inflammation Lower risk of arthritis

Fruits	Vegetables
	Lower risk of diabetes Lower risk of heart disease Cons: Cause digestive symptoms High hunger levels Increase blood sugar levels Weight gain
	Brussels Sprout It is an incredible powerhouse of nutrition. Pros: Fight oxidative stress Protect against bladder Protect against breast cancer Protect against prostate Protect against stomach cancer Protect kidney Protect lungs Reduce inflammation Cons: Gas
	Acorn Squash It is a high-nutritional-value carbohydrate and loaded with vitamins and minerals. Pros: Boosted immune system Improved vision Protection of the skin Strengthening of the bones Cons: Can cause cucurbit poisoning
	Turmeric It contains anti-inflammatory and antioxidant properties, which may offer benefits for human health. Pros: Anti-inflammation Improved Liver Function Increased Antioxidants Lower blood pressure Lower blood sugar Pain Relief Support Brain Health

Fruits	Vegetables
	Support Heart Health
	Cons:
	Acid reflux
	Diarrhea
	Dizziness
	Headaches
	Upset stomach
	Cilantro
	It contains vitamins A-C, and K, and the leaves have folate, potassium, and manganese.
	Pros:
	Protect against body infections
	Protect against illnesses
	Cons:
	Facial swelling
	Hives
	Severe diarrhea
	Stomach pain
	Throat swelling

5 Juicing for Health

5.1 Metabolic wastes

By shifting the blood pH from acid to alkaline, fresh lemon and vegetable juices (green juice, carrot juice, amla juice) aid in the removal of metabolic wastes.

5.2 Constipation

Constipation is a digestive issue that makes regular bowel movements difficult. For such an issue, carrot–beetroot–cucumber juice is indicated. Constipation can be relieved by drinking beet juice on a regular basis. Gout, kidney, and gall bladder disorders can all be helped by combining beetroot and carrot juice. Insoluble fiber is abundant in carrots. Cucumber is a good laxative food as well. It provides bulk to facilitate bowel movement.

5.3 Eyes

Carrot and celery juice include vitamin A, which, according to the Office of Dietary Supplements, influences bone growth, procreation, and cell function in addition to enhancing your eyesight. Carrot and celery juice may help prevent vitamin A deficiency, which can cause symptoms including dry eyes, night blindness, itchy, coarse skin, weak enamel on teeth, and loose stools. Vitamin A also helps to keep the immune system in check.

5.4 Menopause

Menopause is the period of a woman's life during which her ovaries stop producing eggs. Menstruation becomes less frequent and eventually ceases. This is a good time to drink carrot–beetroot–pomegranate juice. Antioxidants are abundant in all three foods, which aid in the fight against the stress brought on by this illness. Pomegranate boosts bone density and has a slew of additional advantages.

5.5 High Blood Pressure (HBP)

A measurement of 140/90 mm Hg or greater is considered high blood pressure. For high blood pressure, carrot juice with garlic is advised. Garlic reduces the risk of cardiovascular disease by lowering blood pressure and cholesterol. Garlic contains chemicals called allicin and hydrogen sulfide, which relax blood vessels and improve blood flow in the arteries.

5.6 Headache

The juice of apples, cucumbers, kale, celery, and ginger is beneficial in the treatment of headaches. Apples have properties that serve to balance the alkaline and acidic levels in the body, reducing headaches, while ginger helps to reduce blood vessel irritation and is commonly used in the treatment of headaches. Cucumbers are abundant in B vitamins, sugar, and electrolytes, and they help prevent headaches by replenishing nutrients lost in the body. Kale is high in magnesium and Omega-3 fatty acids, which migraine sufferers require to avoid attacks, while celery is suggested by many experts for its headache-relieving properties.

5.7 Type 2 Diabetes

Diabetes is a disease that causes elevated blood sugar levels. The key to managing it is to eat the correct foods and exercise regularly. Carrot, Brussel sprout, and bean juices (string beans or French beans) may be beneficial to people with diabetes. Bean pods include diuretic effects. They increase urine flow and aid in the removal of toxins from the body. In addition, brussel sprouts are high in soluble fiber and vitamin C.

5.8 Obesity

Obesity is the mother and cause of the majority of diseases. To stay healthy, one must protect oneself from this condition. A juice made from carrots, cabbage, and green vegetables works well. Green veggies are high in fiber and aid in the elimination of acidic waste. Cabbage juice, on the other hand, inhibits the conversion of carbs to fats, making it useful in the fight against obesity. Carrots are high in carotenoids (antioxidants) and have a high fiber content.

5.9 Cholesterol

Ginger juice can help you lose weight and decrease your cholesterol. When ginger juice is consumed before a meal, it aids digestion. It aids in the elimination of gas and acidity.

5.10 Colds, fevers, and influenza

Vegetable juices, which are abundant in micronutrients and antioxidants, aid in the development of immunity. The perfect formula might be carrot juice blended with oranges, lemon, and garlic. Carotenoids are prevalent in carrots, while vitamin C is rich in oranges and lemons. Garlic is well-known for its antibacterial properties, which make it useful in the treatment of colds\, fever, and flu.

5.11 Pimples and Acne

The best detoxifier for the body is supposed to be neem juice. Antibacterial properties are also present in neem. According to legend, if neem juice were drunk on a daily basis, the skin would remain beautiful, and all ailments will be avoided. Lemon juice mixed with a cup of warm water and consumed first thing in the morning on an empty stomach also help to prevent skin problems.

6 Juicing in pregnancy

Unpasteurized juices might contain dangerous bacteria. To be safe, keep them off the menu. Due to the lack of pasteurization, cold-pressed juice is not suitable for pregnant women.

The trip is to make sure that the place where you buy your fruits and vegetables is careful in how they handle and store their product . It's also critical to wash these products before using them once you bring them home. Organic vegetables are the most significant choice if at all possible.

Another key point to remember is to consume your juice right away. Yes, if kept in the fridge, you can consume it up to 24 hours later. However, it is ideal for preparing enough so that you can drink it right away.

Do you know what Toxoplasma is? This parasite can be found on unwashed fruits and vegetables and is dangerous to both the mother and the unborn child.

Before the sprouts are formed, bacteria can enter into the sprout seeds through breaks in the shell. Once this happens, it's extremely difficult, if not impossible, to get rid of the bacteria. This involves growing and consuming your own sprouts from the comfort of your own home. The contaminated seed has been related to a number of epidemics.

When you create your own juice, you have complete control over how the fruits and vegetables are stored, prepped for juicing, and when the juice is made.

Because many juice bars and restaurants strive to reduce waste, they will frequently use all of the products available in various formats. As a result, some of these establishments selling freshly squeezed juice are not adequately prepared or unpasteurized.

The main concern with unpasteurized juices during pregnancy is that if the fruits and vegetables are not adequately cleaned, pathogens such as salmonella or E. coli may be present, which will make you unwell and may have major consequences for your baby's health.

The most fantastic juice is one that provides you with all of the nutrients you require. Iron, vitamin C-D-E-B6, calcium, folate and beta carotene are just a few of the nutrients, vitamins, and minerals that can be obtained by combining various product .

7   Fruits to Avoid ins pregnancy

During pregnancy, certain fruits must be avoided at all costs.

Grapes
Grapes include a chemical called resveratrol, which has been linked to being hazardous to pregnant women and weakening their digestive systems.

Papaya
Papaya raises your body temperature, which might lead to pregnancy difficulties and even miscarriage.

Pineapple
Bromelain, an enzyme found in pineapples, damages the cervical wall, causing contractions that can lead to a miscarriage.

8   What should I juice?

Carrots are high in beta-carotene and vitamin E.

Kale is high in folate, as well as vitamins K, A, and C. Kale is beneficial in preventing birth abnormalities such as spina bifida.

Fresh ginger root adds a hint of spiciness while also reducing nausea. Ginger is an excellent source of iron and vitamin C.

Beetroot has betacyanin, a potent antioxidant. It boosts energy levels while also acting as an anti-inflammatory.

Tomatoes are abundant in vitamins and antioxidants, which may help with energy and digestion.

Spinach is high in iron and folate, also vitamins A-C, and E. It helps to maintain bone health.

Cucumbers are diuretics that help to reduce edema.

Apple has a lot of vitamin C in it. Apple consumption during pregnancy may lessen the chances of the infant getting asthma and allergies later in life.

Oranges are high in folate, vitamin C, vitamin A, calcium, and thiamin.

Apricots have nutrients that aid in the development and growth of the newborn. Calcium aids in the development of strong bones, and iron helps prevent anemia.
Vitamins A, C, E, and calcium are all present.

Mangoes contains Vitamins A and C. One cup of mango has 100 percentage of a human daily vitamin C need and more than a third of their daily vitamin A requirement.

Pears are high in fiber. Constipation can be alleviated by including enough of fiber in your pregnant diet. Potassium is beneficial to both the mother and the baby's heart health.

Pomegranate may assist in reducing the risk of placental damage, according to research. Vitamin K is also necessary for preserving bone health.

Avocados are high in healthy fats that provide human energy and prevent neural tube abnormalities. They also increase the cells in body that help the growing baby's skin and brain tissues grow.

Guava is high in vitamins C-E, polyphenols, carotenoids, isoflavonoids, and folate, among other nutrients. During pregnancy, guava juice can help relax muscles, aid digestion, and ease constipation.

Bananas are high fiber content can aid with constipation caused by pregnancy. There's some evidence that vitamin B-6 can aid with nausea and vomiting in the first trimester of pregnancy.

Berries are an excellent source of hydration since they are loaded with water. Vitamin C aids iron absorption and help strengthens the immune system.

It would always be best for you if you always inform your doctor about whatever you eat or do during pregnancy. Every human is different, and you may need to avoid some components if you're allergic to them or they're not safe for a pregnant woman.

9   30 Days reboot plan

1-5 Days

Breakfast	1-Snack	Lunch	2-Snack	Dinner
Ingredients cucumber - 1 fresh parsley - 3 springs ginger - 1-inch	Ingredients blueberries - ¼ cup green apple - spinach - 1 handful	Ingredients carrot - ½ lemon - ½ spinach - 1 bunch stalk celery - 1	Ingredients Ginger - ½ -inch Mint - ¼ cup Orange - ¼ cucumber - ¼ Watermelon - ½ cup	Ingredients Apple - 1 Pomegranate - 1 cup
Procedure Procedure All ingredients should be thoroughly washed and dry before juicing. Run each product through the juicer one at a time until all of them are juiced. Serve right away with ice or without ice.	Procedure Procedure All ingredients should be thoroughly washed and dry before juicing. Run each product through the juicer one at a time until all of them are juiced. Serve right away with ice or without ice.	Procedure Procedure All ingredients should be thoroughly washed and dry before juicing. Run each product through the juicer one at a time until all of them are juiced. Serve right away with ice or without ice.	Procedure Procedure All ingredients should be thoroughly washed and dry before juicing. Run each product through the juicer one at a time until all of them are juiced. Serve right away with ice or without ice.	Procedure Procedure All ingredients should be thoroughly washed and dry before juicing. Run each product through the juicer one at a time until all of them are juiced. Serve right away with ice or without ice.
Calories: 56	Calories: 144	Calories: 118	Calories: 75	Calories: 216

6-10 Days

Breakfast	1-Snack	Lunch	2-Snack	Dinner
Ingredients blueberries - ½ cup mint - ¼ cup Strawberries - ½ cup	Ingredients Carrot - ½ Grapefruit - ½ Orange - ½	Ingredients kiwi - 1 orange - ½ pomegranates - ½ cup sweet lime - 1	Ingredients Beetroot - ½ Carrot - ½ Ginger - 1-inch Tomato - ½	Ingredients Ginger - 1-inch Kiwi fruit - 2 Litchis - 6-8
Procedure	Procedure	Procedure	Procedure	Procedure

Breakfast	1-Snack	Lunch	2-Snack	Dinner
All ingredients should be thoroughly washed and dry before juicing. Run each product through the juicer one at a time until all of them are juiced. Serve right away with ice or without ice.	All ingredients should be thoroughly washed and dry before juicing. Run each product through the juicer one at a time until all of them are juiced. Serve right away with ice or without ice.	All ingredients should be thoroughly washed and dry before juicing. Run each product through the juicer one at a time until all of them are juiced. Serve right away with ice or without ice.	All ingredients should be thoroughly washed and dry before juicing. Run each product through the juicer one at a time until all of them are juiced. Serve right away with ice or without ice.	All ingredients should be thoroughly washed and dry before juicing. Run each product through the juicer one at a time until all of them are juiced. Serve right away with ice or without ice.
Calories: 75	Calories: 76	Calories: 152	Calories: 97	Calories: 161

11 15 Days

Breakfast	1-Snack	Lunch	2-Snack	Dinner
Ingredients **Mango - 1** **Avocado - ½** **Figs - 2-3**	Ingredients Orange - 1 Peach - 1	Ingredients Apple - 1 ginger - 1-inch stalks celery - 1	Ingredients beetroot - 1 carrot - 1 fennel bulb - 1/2 lemon - ¼	Ingredients apple - ½ peas - ½ cup Spears asparagus - 2 Spinach - 1 handful
Procedure **All ingredients should be thoroughly washed and dry before juicing. Run each product through the juicer one at a time until all of them are juiced. Serve right away with ice or without ice.**	Procedure All ingredients should be thoroughly washed and dry before juicing. Run each product through the juicer one at a time until all of them are juiced. Serve right away with ice or without ice.	Procedure All ingredients should be thoroughly washed and dry before juicing. Run each product through the juicer one at a time until all of them are juiced. Serve right away with ice or without ice.	Procedure All ingredients should be thoroughly washed and dry before juicing. Run each product through the juicer one at a time until all of them are juiced. Serve right away with ice or without ice.	Procedure All ingredients should be thoroughly washed and dry before juicing. Run each product through the juicer one at a time until all of them are juiced. Serve right away with ice or without ice.
Calories: 518	Calories: 145	Calories: 171	Calories: 86	Calories: 133

16-20 Days

Breakfast	1-Snack	Lunch	2-Snack	Dinner
Ingredients Basil - handful Lime - 1 Mango - 1	Ingredients 1 broccoli head carrot - ¼ coriander - ¼ cup celery sticks - 1 pear - ¼	Ingredients broccoli stalk - 1 carrot - ½ celery stick - 1 Parsley - handful Spinach - 1 handful	Ingredients kiwi - ½ mint leaves - 5 Pear - ½ cucumber - ½ Spinach - 1 handful	Ingredients Apple - 1 Carrot - 1 Kale - handful Spinach - 1 handfuls
Procedure All ingredients should be thoroughly washed and dry before juicing. Run each product through the juicer one at a time until all of them are juiced. Serve right away with ice or without ice.	Procedure All ingredients should be thoroughly washed and dry before juicing. Run each product through the juicer one at a time until all of them are juiced. Serve right away with ice or without ice.	Procedure All ingredients should be thoroughly washed and dry before juicing. Run each product through the juicer one at a time until all of them are juiced. Serve right away with ice or without ice.	Procedure All ingredients should be thoroughly washed and dry before juicing. Run each product through the juicer one at a time until all of them are juiced. Serve right away with ice or without ice.	Procedure All ingredients should be thoroughly washed and dry before juicing. Run each product through the juicer one at a time until all of them are juiced. Serve right away with ice or without ice.
Calories: 229	Calories: 65	Calories: 79	Calories: 98	Calories: 181

21-25 Days

Breakfast	1-Snack	Lunch	2-Snack	Dinner
Ingredients Apple ½ celery stick - 1 cucumber - ½ kale - ½ cup lemon - ¼	Ingredients apple - 1 mint - ½ cup tomato - 1	Ingredients apple - 1 avocado - 1 celery sticks - 3	Ingredients green apple - 1 lime - ½ watermelon - 1 cup	Ingredients beetroot - 1 pear - 1 peas - ½ cup
Procedure All ingredients should be thoroughly	Procedure All ingredients should be thoroughly washed	Procedure All ingredients should be thoroughly washed	Procedure All ingredients should be thoroughly washed	Procedure All ingredients should be thoroughly washed

Breakfast	1-Snack	Lunch	2-Snack	Dinner
washed and dry before juicing. Run each product through the juicer one at a time until all of them are juiced. Serve right away with ice or without ice.	and dry before juicing. Run each product through the juicer one at a time until all of them are juiced. Serve right away with ice or without ice.	and dry before juicing. Run each product through the juicer one at a time until all of them are juiced. Serve right away with ice or without ice.	and dry before juicing. Run each product through the juicer one at a time until all of them are juiced. Serve right away with ice or without ice.	and dry before juicing. Run each product through the juicer one at a time until all of them are juiced. Serve right away with ice or without ice.
Calories: 98	Calories: 147	Calories: 424	Calories: 165	Calories: 161

26-30 Days

Breakfast	1-Snack	Lunch	2-Snack	Dinner
Ingredients Avocado - 1 blackberries - ½ cup mint - ½ cup Peach - 1 spinach - 1 cup	Ingredients beetroot - ¼ blueberries - ½ cup mint ¼ cup spinach - 1 cup	Ingredients fennel bulb - ½ kale - ½ cup lemon - ½ orange - 1 pear - 1	Ingredients avocado - 1 Lemon juice - 1 raspberries - ½ cup strawberries - ½ cup	Ingredients guava - 1 lemon - ½ mango - 1 cup Spinach - ½ cup
Procedure All ingredients should be thoroughly washed and dry before juicing. Run each product through the juicer one at a time until all of them are juiced. Serve right away with ice or without ice.	Procedure All ingredients should be thoroughly washed and dry before juicing. Run each product through the juicer one at a time until all of them are juiced. Serve right away with ice or without ice.	Procedure All ingredients should be thoroughly washed and dry before juicing. Run each product through the juicer one at a time until all of them are juiced. Serve right away with ice or without ice.	Procedure All ingredients should be thoroughly washed and dry before juicing. Run each product through the juicer one at a time until all of them are juiced. Serve right away with ice or without ice.	Procedure All ingredients should be thoroughly washed and dry before juicing. Run each product through the juicer one at a time until all of them are juiced. Serve right away with ice or without ice.
Calories: 396	Calories: 68	Calories: 223	Calories: 348	Calories: 168

10 Morning Juices

Morning juices could be made from fruits, green vegetables, berries, and herbs. These contain the vitamins, minerals, and nutrients that the majority of people require and may be prepared in 5 minutes for a delightful drink. The fibre in most morning juices can help you control your bowel motions and eliminate pollutants. They're delicious and help to brighten up the mornings.

10.1 Carrot Juice

Prep Time: 5 minutes | Cook Time: 0 minutes | Servings: 4

INGREDIENTS
carrots - 6
stalks celery - 6
apple Ambrosia - 2
lime wedge - 1
fresh ginger - 1-inch

PROCEDURE
All ingredients should be thoroughly washed and dry before juicing.
Run each product through the juicer one at a time until all of them are juiced.
Serve right away with ice or without ice.

Nutrition facts: [per serving]
Calories: 85 | fat 0.5g | carbs 21g | protein 2g | sugar 30g

10.2 Good Morning Juice

Prep Time: 5 minutes | Cook Time: 0 minutes | Servings: 2

INGREDIENTS
cucumber with skin on - 1
handful spinach - 1handful
celery stalks - 8
lime - 1
lemon - 1
fresh ginger - 1-inch

PROCEDURE
All ingredients should be thoroughly washed and dry before juicing.
Run each product through the juicer one at a time until all of them are juiced.
Serve right away with ice or without ice.

Nutrition facts: [per serving]
Calories: 54 | fat 0.5g | carbs 11.2g | protein 2.6g | sugar 4.8g

10.3 Sweet Potato, Carrot and Orange Juice

Prep Time: 5 minutes | Cook Time: 0 minutes | Servings: 3

INGREDIENTS
sweet potatoes, peeled - 2
carrots - 3
apples - 3
oranges - 4
fresh ginger - 1-nch

PROCEDURE
All ingredients should be thoroughly washed and dry before juicing.
Run each product through the juicer one at a time until all of them are juiced.
Serve right away with ice or without ice.

Nutrition facts: [per serving]
Calories: 328 | fat 0.9g | carbs 81.7g | protein 4.2g | sugar 41.7g

10.4 Pineapple Surprise Juice

Prep Time: 5 minutes | Cook Time: 0 minutes | Servings: 4

INGREDIENTS

Pineapple, peeled - 1
carrots - 4
apple - 1
lemon - 1
lime - 1

PROCEDURE

All ingredients should be thoroughly washed and dry before juicing.
Run each product through the juicer one at a time until all of them are juiced.
Serve right away with ice or without ice.

NUTRITION FACTS: [PER SERVING]

Calories: 173 | fat 0.5g | carbs 44.5g | protein 2.1g | sugar 31.7g

10.5   Root Juice

Prep Time: 5 minutes | Cook Time: 0 minutes | Servings: 2

INGREDIENTS

beetroot, peeled - 1
carrots - 1
pineapple - 1 cup
lemon - 1

PROCEDURE

All ingredients should be thoroughly washed and dry before juicing.
Run each product through the juicer one at a time until all of them are juiced.
Serve right away with ice or without ice.

NUTRITION FACTS: [PER SERVING]

Calories: 111 | fat 0g | carbs 19g | protein 1g | sugar 7g

10.6   Harvest Juice

Prep Time: 5 minutes | Cook Time: 0 minutes | Servings: 4

INGREDIENTS

apples - 3
pears - 3
blood oranges – 3
fresh cranberries - 2 cup

PROCEDURE

All ingredients should be thoroughly washed and dry before juicing.
Run each product through the juicer one at a time until all of them are juiced.
Serve right away with ice or without ice.

NUTRITION FACTS: [PER SERVING]

Calories: 273 | fat 0.7g | carbs 68.2g | protein 2.3g | sugar 47.6g

10.7   Celap Juice

Prep Time: 5 minutes | Cook Time: 0 minutes | Servings: 2

INGREDIENTS

stalks celery - 1-12
apple - 1
fresh ginger - 1-inch
lemon - ¼

PROCEDURE

All ingredients should be thoroughly washed and dry before juicing.
Run each product through the juicer one at a time until all of them are juiced.
Serve right away with ice or without ice.

NUTRITION FACTS: [PER SERVING]

Calories: 87 | fat 0.6g | carbs 21g | protein 1.3g | sugar 13g

10.8 Cater Juice

Prep Time: 10 minutes | Cook Time: 0 minutes | Servings: 1

INGREDIENTS
beet - 1
apple - 1
ginger - 1-inch
carrots - 3

PROCEDURE
All ingredients should be thoroughly washed and dry before juicing.
Run each product through the juicer one at a time until all of them are juiced.
Serve right away with ice or without ice.

NUTRITION FACTS: [PER SERVING]
Calories: 254 | fat 0.9g | carbs 62.6g | protein 4.3g | sugar 40.3g

10.9 Granny Juice

Prep Time: 10 minutes | Cook Time: 0 minutes | Servings: 4

INGREDIENTS
curly kale - 1 bunch
lemon - 1
fresh ginger - 1-inch
cucumber - 1
granny smith apples - 2
celery stalks, whole - 4

PROCEDURE
All ingredients should be thoroughly washed and dry before juicing.
Run each product through the juicer one at a time until all of them are juiced.
Serve right away with ice or without ice.

NUTRITION FACTS: [PER SERVING]
Calories: 84 | fat 0.4g | carbs 21.7g | protein 1.6g | sugar 13.4g

10.10 Blue Gala Juice

Prep Time: 5 minutes | Cook Time: 0 minutes | Servings: 3

INGREDIENTS
gala apples - 2
carrots - 2
orange - 1
kale leaves - 3-4
blackberries - 1 cup

PROCEDURE
All ingredients should be thoroughly washed and dry before juicing.
Run each product through the juicer one at a time until all of them are juiced.
Serve right away with ice or without ice.

NUTRITION FACTS: [PER SERVING]
Calories: 116 | fat 0.7g | carbs 27.1g | protein 1.9g | sugar 19.4g

10.11 Spin Juice

Prep Time: 5 minutes | Cook Time: 0 minutes | Servings: 2

INGREDIENTS
strawberries - 3
apples - 3
carrots - 3
spinach - 1 cup

PROCEDURE
All ingredients should be thoroughly washed and dry before juicing.
Run each product through the juicer one at a time until all of them are juiced.
Serve right away with ice or without ice.

NUTRITION FACTS: [PER SERVING]
Calories: 221 | fat 0.7g | carbs 57.1g | protein 2.2g | sugar 40.2g

10.12 Awi Juice

Prep Time: 5 minutes | Cook Time: 0 minutes | Servings: 2

INGREDIENTS

apples - 2
kiwis - 1
mint leaves - ½ cup
lemon - 1

PROCEDURE

All ingredients should be thoroughly washed and dry before juicing.
Run each product through the juicer one at a time until all of them are juiced.
Serve right away with ice or without ice.

NUTRITION FACTS: [PER SERVING]

Calories: 217 | fat 1.5g | carbs 53.9g | protein 2.7g | sugar 37.5g

10.13 Pach Juice

Prep Time: 5 minutes | Cook Time: 0 minutes | Servings: 2

INGREDIENTS

peaches - 2
apricots - 2
apples - 2

PROCEDURE

All ingredients should be thoroughly washed and dry before juicing.
Run each product through the juicer one at a time until all of them are juiced.
Serve right away with ice or without ice.

NUTRITION FACTS: [per serving]

Calories: 192 | fat 1g | carbs 48.6g | protein 2.5g | sugar 40.4g

10.14 Rock Juice

Prep Time: 5 minutes | Cook Time: 0 minutes | Servings: 3

INGREDIENTS

rock melon - ½
oranges - 4
pears - 2
lime - ½

PROCEDURE

All ingredients should be thoroughly washed and dry before juicing.
Run each product through the juicer one at a time until all of them are juiced.
Serve right away with ice or without ice.

NUTRITION FACTS: [PER SERVING]

Calories: 243 | fat 0.8g | carbs 61.5g | protein 4g | sugar 47.3g

10.15 Cucap Juice

Prep Time: 5 minutes | Cook Time: 0 minutes | Servings: 3

INGREDIENTS

oranges - 3
fresh ginger - 1-inch
red apples - 2
cucumbers - 2
fresh pineapple chunks - 1 cup

PROCEDURE

All ingredients should be thoroughly washed and dry before juicing.
Run each product through the juicer one at a time until all of them are juiced.
Serve right away with ice or without ice.

Nutrition facts: [per serving]

Calories: 194 | fat 0.7g | carbs 49.7g | protein 3.2g | sugar 35.7g

11 Fruit-Based Juices

Fruit juice is 100 % pure juice prepared from fresh fruit flesh or whole fruit, depending on the variety. Sugars, sweeteners, preservatives, flavorings, and colorings are not authorized in fruit juice. Fresh juices are high in vitamins and antioxidants, which are beneficial to human health.

11.1 Big Black Juice

Prep Time: 5 minutes | Cook Time: 0 minutes | Servings: 1

INGREDIENTS
orange - 1
apple - 1
black grapes - ½ cup
kiwi - 1

PROCEDURE
All ingredients should be thoroughly washed and dry before juicing.
Run each product through the juicer one at a time until all of them are juiced.
Serve right away with ice or without ice.

NUTRITION PER SERVING:
Calories: 280 | fat 1.2g | carbs 71.5g | protein 3.5g | sugar 54.7g

11.2 Pomes Juice

Prep Time: 10 minutes | Cook Time: 0 minutes | Servings: 2

INGREDIENTS
Oranges - 2
Grapes - 1 cup
Pomegranate - 1
apple - 1
kiwi - 1
Lemon -1

PROCEDURE
All ingredients should be thoroughly washed and dry before juicing.
Run each product through the juicer one at a time until all of them are juiced.
Serve right away with ice or without ice.

NUTRITION PER SERVING:
Calories: 251 | fat 0.8g | carbs 64.2g | protein 3.3g | sugar 50.4g

11.3 Pineberry Juice

Prep Time: 10 minutes | Cook Time: 0 minutes | Servings: 3

INGREDIENTS
pineapple - 1 cup
green apple - 1
orange - 2
grapes - 1 cup
strawberry - 6

PROCEDURE
All ingredients should be thoroughly washed and dry before juicing.
Run each product through the juicer one at a time until all of them are juiced.
Serve right away with ice or without ice.

Nutrition per serving:
Calories: 152 | fat 0.5g | carbs 39g | protein 2g | sugar 30.8g

11.4 Plum Juice

Prep Time: 5 minutes | Cook Time: 0 minutes | Servings: 2

INGREDIENTS
plum - 4

pineapple - 2 cups

PROCEDURE

All ingredients should be thoroughly washed and dry before juicing.

Run each product through the juicer one at a time until all of them are juiced.

Serve right away with ice or without ice.

NUTRITION PER SERVING:

Calories: 142 | fat 0.6g | carbs 37.7g | protein 1.9g | sugar 30.3g

11.5   Pomberry Juice

Prep Time: 10 minutes | Cook Time: 0 minutes | Servings: 2

INGREDIENTS

pomegranate seeds - 2 cups
strawberry - 6

PROCEDURE

All ingredients should be thoroughly washed and dry before juicing.

Run each product through the juicer one at a time until all of them are juiced.

Serve right away with ice or without ice.

NUTRITION PER SERVING:

Calories112 | fat 0.1g | carbs 26.8g | protein 1.2g | sugar 13.8g

11.6   Aplime Juice

Prep Time: 10 minutes | Cook Time: 0 minutes | Servings: 4

INGREDIENTS

pineapple - 1
apples - 2
oranges - 2
pears - 2
lime - 1

PROCEDURE

All ingredients should be thoroughly washed and dry before juicing.

Run each product through the juicer one at a time until all of them are juiced.

Serve right away with ice or without ice.

NUTRITION PER SERVING:

Calories: 247 | fat 1g | carbs 65g | protein 3g | sugar 47g

11.7   Rapna Juice

Prep Time: 10 minutes | Cook Time: 0 minutes | Servings: 4

INGREDIENTS

pineapple - 2 cups
orange - 1
banana - 1
apple - 1
strawberries - 1 cup
grapes - 1 cup

PROCEDURE

All ingredients should be thoroughly washed and dry before juicing.

Run each product through the juicer one at a time until all of them are juiced.

Serve right away with ice or without ice.

NUTRITION PER SERVING:

Calories: 145 | fat 0.6g | carbs 37.4g | protein 1.7g | sugar 27.3g

11.8   Tangle Juice

Prep Time: 5 minutes | Cook Time: 0 minutes | Servings: 1

INGREDIENTS

apple - 1
tangerine - 1
Lemon - 1

PROCEDURE

All ingredients should be thoroughly washed and dry before juicing.

Run each product through the juicer one at a time until all of them are juiced.

Serve right away with ice or without ice.

NUTRITION PER SERVING:

Calories165 | fat 0.7g | carbs 43.4g | protein 1.5g | sugar 32.5g

11.9 Sapay Juice

Prep Time: 10 minutes | Cook Time: 0 minutes | Servings: 1

INGREDIENTS

Papaya - ½ cup

Pomegranate - ½ cup

Guava -1

Sapota - 1

PROCEDURE

All ingredients should be thoroughly washed and dry before juicing.

Run each product through the juicer one at a time until all of them are juiced.

Serve right away with ice or without ice.

NUTRITION PER SERVING:

Calories: 248 | fat 1.1g | carbs 58.4g | protein 4.5g | sugar 46.1g

11.10 Passion Juice

Prep Time: 5 minutes | Cook Time: 0 minutes | Servings: 1

INGREDIENTS

Mango - 1

Passion fruits - 2

PROCEDURE

All ingredients should be thoroughly washed and dry before juicing.

Run each product through the juicer one at a time until all of them are juiced.

Serve right away with ice or without ice.

NUTRITION PER SERVING:

Calories: 237 | fat 1.5g | carbs 58.6g | protein 3.6g | sugar 49.9g

11.11 Range Juice

Prep Time: 10 minutes | Cook Time: 0 minutes | Servings: 1

INGREDIENTS

Orange - 1

Pineapple - ½ cup

lemon - ½

PROCEDURE

All ingredients should be thoroughly washed and dry before juicing.

Run each product through the juicer one at a time until all of them are juiced.

Serve right away with ice or without ice.

NUTRITION PER SERVING:

Calories: 145 | fat 0.4g | carbs 39.8g | protein 2.6g | sugar 30.2g

11.12 Mano Juice

Prep Time: 10 minutes | Cook Time: 0 minutes | Servings: 2

INGREDIENTS

mangoes - 4

orange - 1

lemon - 1

PROCEDURE

All ingredients should be thoroughly washed and dry before juicing.

Run each product through the juicer one at a time until all of them are juiced.

Serve right away with ice or without ice.

NUTRITION PER SERVING:
Calories: 448 | fat 2.7g | carbs 112g | protein 6.4g | sugar 100.5g

11.13 Ranp Juice

Prep Time: 5 minutes | Cook Time: 0 minutes | Servings: 1

INGREDIENTS
oranges - 2
papaya - 1 cup

PROCEDURE
All ingredients should be thoroughly washed and dry before juicing.
Run each product through the juicer one at a time until all of them are juiced.
Serve right away with ice or without ice.

NUTRITION PER SERVING:
Calories: 235 | fat 0.8g | carbs 58.8g | protein 4.2g | sugar 54.7g

11.14 Cherry Juice

Prep Time: 5 minutes | Cook Time: 0 minutes | Servings: 1

INGREDIENTS
Mango - 1

cherry - ½ cup
dragon fruit - ½

PROCEDURE
All ingredients should be thoroughly washed and dry before juicing.
Run each product through the juicer one at a time until all of them are juiced.
Serve right away with ice or without ice.

NUTRITION PER SERVING:
Calories: 249 | fat 1.6g | carbs 61.9g | protein 3.8g | sugar 53.4g

11.15 Dew Juice

Prep Time: 5 minutes | Cook Time: 0 minutes | Servings: 1

INGREDIENTS
Honeydew - 1 cup
green apple - 2

PROCEDURE
All ingredients should be thoroughly washed and dry before juicing.
Run each product through the juicer one at a time until all of them are juiced.
Serve right away with ice or without ice.

NUTRITION PER SERVING:
Calories: 293 | fat 1g | carbs 77.1g | protein 2.1g | sugar 60.2g

12 Vegetable-Based Juices

Juices are prepared from a variety of vegetables blended together and served for breakfast, snacks, or any other time. It contains no sugar. Vegetable juice has the ability to improve nutrient absorption, protect the heart, promote hydration, minimize hair loss, detoxify the body, lower your risk of chronic disease, support skin health, increase circulation, and strengthen the immune system, among other things.

12.1 Chito Juice

Prep Time: 5 minutes | Cook Time: 0 minutes | Servings: 2

INGREDIENTS
Chives - ¼ cup
Tomatoes - 2
fresh Jalapeño, seeded - ¼
red Bell pepper - 1
stalks Celery - 2
Carrot - 1

PROCEDURE
All ingredients should be thoroughly washed and dry before juicing.
Run each product through the juicer one at a time until all of them are juiced.
Serve right away with ice or without ice.

NUTRITION PER SERVING:
Calories: 46 | fat 0.5g | carbs 9g | protein 1g | sugar 7g

12.2 Rooter Juice

Prep Time: 10 minutes | Cook Time: 0 minutes | Servings: 1

INGREDIENTS
Carrot - 1
Beetroot - ½
Tomato - ½
Ginger - 1-inch
Mint - 1 spring

PROCEDURE
All ingredients should be thoroughly washed and dry before juicing.
Run each product through the juicer one at a time until all of them are juiced.
Serve right away with ice or without ice.

NUTRITION PER SERVING:
Calories: 69 | fat 0.4g | carbs 15.4g | protein 2.4g | sugar 8.1g

12.3 Pepper Juice

Prep Time: 10 minutes | Cook Time: 0 minutes | Servings: 7

INGREDIENTS
tomatoes - 5 pounds
green pepper - ¼ cup
carrot - ¼ cup
celery ¼ cup
lemon juice - ¼ cup
onion - 2 tbsp.
serrano peppers - 1

PROCEDURE
All ingredients should be thoroughly washed and dry before juicing.
Run each product through the juicer one at a time until all of them are juiced.
Serve right away with ice or without ice.

NUTRITION PER SERVING:
Calories: 66 | fat 1g | carbs 15g | protein 3g | sugar 9g

12.4 Pap Juice

Prep Time: 10 minutes | Cook Time: 0 minutes | Servings: 1

INGREDIENTS

Carrot - ½
Papaya - 4 cubes
Lettuce - 2 leaves
Tomato - ½
lemon - ½

PROCEDURE

All ingredients should be thoroughly washed and dry before juicing.
Run each product through the juicer one at a time until all of them are juiced.
Serve right away with ice or without ice.

NUTRITION PER SERVING:

Calories50 | fat 0.3g | carbs 12.6g | protein 1g | sugar 7.6g

12.5 Leafy Juice

Prep Time: 10 minutes | Cook Time: 0 minutes | Servings: 2

INGREDIENTS

celery stalks – 4
cucumber - ½
parsley leaf - 1 bunch
kale leaves - 3
baby spinach - ½ handful
lime - 1

PROCEDURE

All ingredients should be thoroughly washed and dry before juicing.
Run each product through the juicer one at a time until all of them are juiced.
Serve right away with ice or without ice.

NUTRITION PER SERVING:

Calories: 32 | fat 0.3g | carbs 7.4g | protein 1.7g | sugar 2.1g

12.6 Stak Juice

Prep Time: 5 minutes | Cook Time: 0 minutes | Servings: 1

INGREDIENTS

Tomatoes - 2
stalk Celery - ½
Cucumber - ½
Parsley - 1 handful

PROCEDURE

All ingredients should be thoroughly washed and dry before juicing.
Run each product through the juicer one at a time until all of them are juiced.
Serve right away with ice or without ice.

NUTRITION PER SERVING:

Calories: 90 | fat 1.1g | carbs 19.1g | protein 5g | sugar 9.6g

12.7 Tober Juice

Prep Time: 5 minutes | Cook Time: 0 minutes | Servings: 1

INGREDIENTS

carrot - 1
tomato - 1
cucumber - ½

PROCEDURE

All ingredients should be thoroughly washed and dry before juicing.
Run each product through the juicer one at a time until all of them are juiced.
Serve right away with ice or without ice.

NUTRITION PER SERVING:

Calories: 70 | fat 0.4g | carbs 16.2g | protein 2.6g | sugar 8.7g

12.8 Red Rush Juice

Prep Time: 5 minutes | Cook Time: 0 minutes | Servings: 1

INGREDIENTS
Carrot - 1
Tomato - 1
Mint leaves - 1 cup
Lemon - 1

PROCEDURE
All ingredients should be thoroughly washed and dry before juicing.
Run each product through the juicer one at a time until all of them are juiced.
Serve right away with ice or without ice on.

NUTRITION PER SERVING:
Calories: 96 | fat 0.8g | carbs 21.3g | protein 4.9g | sugar 7g

12.9 Clove Juice

Prep Time: 5 minutes | Cook Time: 0 minutes | Servings: 2

INGREDIENTS
cucumbers - ½
tomatoes - 4
kale - ½ bunch
basil - ½ bunch
garlic clove - 1

PROCEDURE
All ingredients should be thoroughly washed and dry before juicing.
Run each product through the juicer one at a time until all of them are juiced.
Serve right away with ice or without ice.

NUTRITION PER SERVING:
Calories: 67 | fat 0.6g | carbs 14.7g | protein 3.4g | sugar 7.8g

12.10 Ground Juice

Prep Time: 5 minutes | Cook Time: 0 minutes | Servings: 2

INGREDIENTS
tomatoes - 2
bottle ground - 2
ginger - 1-inch

PROCEDURE
All ingredients should be thoroughly washed and dry before juicing.
Run each product through the juicer one at a time until all of them are juiced.
Serve right away with ice or without ice.

NUTRITION PER SERVING:
Calories: 52 | fat 0.7g | carbs 11.1g | protein 1.9g | sugar 3.5g

12.11 Lak Juice

Prep Time: 5 minutes | Cook Time: 0 minutes | Servings: 2

INGREDIENTS
Celery stalks - 2
Carrots - 2
Tomato - 1
Kale - ½ bunch

PROCEDURE
All ingredients should be thoroughly washed and dry before juicing.
Run each product through the juicer one at a time until all of them are juiced.
Serve right away with ice or without ice.

NUTRITION PER SERVING:
Calories: 42 | fat 1g | carbs 9.5g | protein 1.4g | sugar 4.1g

12.12 Dark Juice

Prep Time: 5 minutes | Cook Time: 0 minutes | Servings: 1

INGREDIENTS
Cucumber - 1 ½
Spinach - 1 cup

PROCEDURE
All ingredients should be thoroughly washed and dry before juicing.
Run each product through the juicer one at a time until all of them are juiced.
Serve right away with ice or without ice.

NUTRITION PER SERVING:
Calories: 75 | fat 0.6g | carbs 17.5g | protein 3.8g | sugar 7.7g

12.13 Troot Juice

Prep Time: 5 minutes | Cook Time: 0 minutes | Servings: 1

INGREDIENTS
carrot - ¼
Beetroot - ¼
stalks Celery - 1
mint leaves - 1 cup

PROCEDURE
All ingredients should be thoroughly washed and dry before juicing.
Run each product through the juicer one at a time until all of them are juiced.
Serve right away with ice or without ice.

NUTRITION PER SERVING:
Calories: 27 | fat 0.2g | carbs 5.7g | protein 1.3g | sugar 2.4g

12.14 Darkish Juice

Prep Time: 5 minutes | Cook Time: 0 minutes | Servings: 1

INGREDIENTS
Mint - 1 cup
Cucumber - 1
Broccoli - 1 cup

PROCEDURE
All ingredients should be thoroughly washed and dry before juicing.
Run each product through the juicer one at a time until all of them are juiced.
Serve right away with ice or without ice.

NUTRITION PER SERVING:
Calories: 116 | fat .3g | carbs 24.6g | protein 7.5g | sugar 6.6g

12.15 Cum Juice

Prep Time: 5 minutes | Cook Time: 0 minutes | Servings: 1

INGREDIENTS
lemon - 1
Ginger - 1-inch
Parsley - ½ cup
Cucumber - 1

PROCEDURE
All ingredients should be thoroughly washed and dry before juicing.
Run each product through the juicer one at a time until all of them are juiced.
Serve right away with ice or without ice.

NUTRITION PER SERVING:
Calories: 125 | fat 1.6g | carbs 28.9g | protein 4.9g | sugar 7.3g

13 Green Juices

Green juices are made with different green vegetables and fruits such as kale, celery, swiss chard, spinach, wheatgrass, parsley, green apple, green grapes, and mint. Fresh green juice consumption can help to reduce inflammation, boost heart and brain health, and promote good digestion. Juicing can also help certain populations heal faster in the short term.

13.1 Evergreen Juice

Prep Time: 10 minutes | Cook Time: 0 minutes | Servings: 2

INGREDIENTS
fresh parsley - ½ cup
spinach - 3 cups
lemon, peeled - ½
pears - 2
stalks celery, trimmed - 6

PROCEDURE
All ingredients should be thoroughly washed and dry before juicing.
Run each product through the juicer one at a time until all of them are juiced.
Serve right away with ice or without ice.

NUTRITION PER SERVING:
Calories: 91 | fat 1g | carbs 20g | protein 1g | sugar 15g

13.2 Apple Spinach Juice

Prep Time: 10 minutes | Cook Time: 0 minutes | Servings: 2

INGREDIENTS
spinach - 1 ¼ cup
grapefruit - ½
green apples - 2
fresh ginger - 1-inch
stalks celery - 2

PROCEDURE

All ingredients should be thoroughly washed and dry before juicing.
Run each product through the juicer one at a time until all of them are juiced.
Serve right away with ice or without ice.

NUTRITION PER SERVING:
Calories: 55 | fat 0.5g | carbs 13g | protein 1g | sugar 10g

13.3 Green Spinach Juice

Prep Time: 10 minutes | Cook Time: 0 minutes | Servings: 2

INGREDIENTS
pears - 2
spinach - 2 handfuls
stalk celery - 1
ginger - ½ -inch
fennel bulb - ¼

PROCEDURE
All ingredients should be thoroughly washed and dry before juicing.
Run each product through the juicer one at a time until all of them are juiced.
Serve right away with ice or without ice.

NUTRITION PER SERVING:
Calories: 139 | fat 0.3g | carbs 33.0g | protein 1.8g | sugar 20.7g

13.4 Kale Juice

Prep Time: 10 minutes | Cook Time: 0 minutes | Servings: 1

INGREDIENTS

kale leaves - 2

head of romaine lettuce - 1

parsley - handful

Granny Smith apple - 1

lemons - 2

PROCEDURE

All ingredients should be thoroughly washed and dry before juicing.

Run each product through the juicer one at a time until all of them are juiced.

Serve right away with ice or without ice.

NUTRITION PER SERVING:

Calories: 189 | fat 1g | carbs 38g | protein 7g | sugar 16g

13.5 Neel Juice

Prep Time: 5 minutes | Cook Time: 0 minutes | Servings: 1

INGREDIENTS

celery stick - 1

kale - 2 handfuls

fennel - ¼

fresh ginger - ½ -inch

pears - 2

PROCEDURE

All ingredients should be thoroughly washed and dry before juicing.

Run each product through the juicer one at a time until all of them are juiced.

Serve right away with ice or without ice.

Nutrition per serving:

Calories: 237 | fat 0.7g | carbs 60.4g | protein 3.3g | sugar 32.6g

13.6 Swiss Juice

Prep Time: 10 minutes | Cook Time: 0 minutes | Servings: 4

INGREDIENTS

apples - 6

oranges - 2

cups Swiss chard - 4 cups

celery stalks - 2

PROCEDURE

All ingredients should be thoroughly washed and dry before juicing.

Run each product through the juicer one at a time until all of them are juiced.

Serve right away with ice or without ice.

Nutrition per serving:

Calories: 229 | fat 0.9g | carbs 59.3g | protein 2.6g | sugar 44.2g

13.7 Ach Juice

Prep Time: 10 minutes | Cook Time: 0 minutes | Servings: 1

INGREDIENTS

spinach - 1 cup

apples, diced - ½ cup

watermelon - ½

PROCEDURE

All ingredients should be thoroughly washed and dry before juicing.

Run each product through the juicer one at a time until all of them are juiced.

Serve right away with ice or without ice.

NUTRITION PER SERVING:

Calories: 83 | fat 0.4g | carbs 21.1g | protein 1.5g | sugar 15.5g

13.8 Ramber Juice

Prep Time: 5 minutes | Cook Time: 0 minutes | Servings: 1

INGREDIENTS

kale - 1 cup

orange - 1

celery stalks - 3

cucumber - ½

lemon juice - ½

PROCEDURE

All ingredients should be thoroughly washed and dry before juicing.

Run each product through the juicer one at a time until all of them are juiced.

Serve right away with ice or without ice.

NUTRITION PER SERVING:

Calories: 158 | fat 0.7g | carbs 36.2g | protein 5.3g | sugar 21g

13.9 Coli Juice

Prep Time: 10 minutes | Cook Time: 0 minutes | Servings: 2

INGREDIENTS

celery stalks - 4

carrot - 1

broccoli - 2 cups

apple - 1

lemon - ½

PROCEDURE

All ingredients should be thoroughly washed and dry before juicing.

Run each product through the juicer one at a time until all of them are juiced.

Serve right away with ice or without ice.

NUTRITION PER SERVING:

Calories: 126 | fat 0.8g | carbs 28.6g | protein 4.1g | sugar 16.7g

13.10 Berle Juice

Prep Time: 10 minutes | Cook Time: 0 minutes | Servings: 2

INGREDIENTS

strawberries - 10

celery stalks - 2

green apple - 1

cucumber - 1

PROCEDURE

All ingredients should be thoroughly washed and dry before juicing.

Run each product through the juicer one at a time until all of them are juiced.

Serve right away with ice or without ice.

NUTRITION PER SERVING:

Calories: 130 | fat 0.9g | carbs 32.1g | protein 2.6g | sugar 20.9g

13.11 Gin Juice

Prep Time: 10 minutes | Cook Time: 0 minutes | Servings: 3

INGREDIENTS

fresh ginger - 1-inch

spinach - 1 cup

celery stalks - 3

apples - 3

pear - 2

cucumber - 1

lemon - 1

PROCEDURE

All ingredients should be thoroughly washed and dry before juicing.

Run each product through the juicer one at a time until all of them are juiced.

Serve right away with ice or without ice.

NUTRITION PER SERVING:

Calories: 196 | fat 0.9g | carbs 50.1g | protein 2.2g | sugar 34.7g

13.12 Pin Juice

Prep Time: 5 minutes | Cook Time: 0 minutes | Servings: 1

INGREDIENTS

pineapple - 1 cup
kale leaves - 5
cucumber - 1
lemon - 1

PROCEDURE

All ingredients should be thoroughly washed and dry before juicing.
Run each product through the juicer one at a time until all of them are juiced.
Serve right away with ice or without ice.

NUTRITION PER SERVING:

Calories: 97 | fat 0.9g | carbs 19.7g | protein 4.6g | sugar 6.7g

13.13 Limle Juice

Prep Time: 5 minutes | Cook Time: 0 minutes | Servings: 1

INGREDIENTS

Lime - ½
apples - 2
kale - handful
jalapeno - 1
fresh ginger - ½ inch

PROCEDURE

All ingredients should be thoroughly washed and dry before juicing.
Run each product through the juicer one at a time until all of them are juiced.
Serve right away with ice or without ice.

NUTRITION PER SERVING:

Calories: 275 | fat 0.9g | carbs 71g | protein 3.5g | sugar 47.2g

13.14 Tuce juice

Prep Time: 10 minutes | Cook Time: 0 minutes | Servings: 2

INGREDIENTS

head lettuce - 1
cucumber - 1
spinach - ½ cup
kale leaves - 3
lime - ½
green apples - 3

PROCEDURE

All ingredients should be thoroughly washed and dry before juicing.
Run each product through the juicer one at a time until all of them are juiced.
Serve right away with ice or without ice.

NUTRITION PER SERVING:

Calories: 231 | fat 1.1g | carbs 59.5g | protein 3.4g | sugar 39.2g

13.15 Chard Juice

Prep Time: 10 minutes | Cook Time: 0 minutes | Servings: 2

INGREDIENTS

Swiss chard leaves - 3
parsley - 1 cup
apples - 2
oranges - 2
cucumber - ½
spinach - ½ cup

PROCEDURE

All ingredients should be thoroughly washed and dry before juicing.
Run each product through the juicer one at a time until all of them are juiced.
Serve right away with ice or without ice.

NUTRITION PER SERVING:

Calories: 240 | fat 1.2g | carbs 60g | protein 5.2g | sugar 42.8g

14 Brain-nourishing Juices

These juices are high in potassium, which aids with brain health. Potassium enables nerve cells in your brain to send nerve impulses that are made up of brief electrical bursts. These impulses carry data between your brain cells, which is necessary for brain function. Polyphenol plant components in juices may have brain-nourishing properties. Nootropics are a type of natural or synthetic compound that can help you think more clearly. These drinks are high in polyphenol and nootropic components, which aid in nourishing the brain.

14.1 Broles Juice

Prep Time: 4 minutes | Cook Time: 0 minutes | Servings: 2

INGREDIENTS
Broccoli - 1 cup
Apples - 3
Garlic clove - 1

PROCEDURE
All ingredients should be thoroughly washed and dry before juicing.
Run each product through the juicer one at a time until all of them are juiced.
Serve right away with ice or without ice.

NUTRITION PER SERVING:
Calories: 192 | fat 0.8g | carbs 49.7g | protein 2.3g | sugar 35.6g

14.2 Pincar Juice

Prep Time: 10 minutes | Cook Time: 0 minutes | Servings: 2

INGREDIENTS
Apple - 1 cup
Beetroot - ¼ cup
Carrot - 1 ½ cup
Spinach - ½

PROCEDURE
All ingredients should be thoroughly washed and dry before juicing.

Run each product through the juicer one at a time until all of them are juiced.
Serve right away with ice or without ice.

NUTRITION PER SERVING:
Calories: 103 | fat 0.3g | carbs 25.9g | protein 1.6g | sugar 17.4g

14.3 Gap Juice

Prep Time: 10 minutes | Cook Time: 0 minutes | Servings: 4

INGREDIENTS

Red Grapes - 4 cups
spinach - 1 ½ cup
Brussels sprouts - 1 cup

PROCEDURE
All ingredients should be thoroughly washed and dry before juicing.
Run each product through the juicer one at a time until all of them are juiced.
Serve right away with ice or without ice.

NUTRITION PER SERVING:

Calories: 116 | fat 0.1g | carbs 29.4g | protein 2.1g | sugar 23.5g

14.4 Acorn Juice

Prep Time: 10 minutes | Cook Time: 0 minutes | Servings: 4

INGREDIENTS

Carrots - 4
Acorn squash - ¼
pineapple - 2 cups

PROCEDURE

All ingredients should be thoroughly washed and dry before juicing.
Run each product through the juicer one at a time until all of them are juiced.
Serve right away with ice or without ice.

NUTRITION PER SERVING:

Calories: 77 | fat 0.1g | carbs 19.6g | protein 1.2g | sugar 11.1g

14.5 Peen Juice

Prep Time: 10 minutes | Cook Time: 0 minutes | Servings: 2

INGREDIENTS

Green peas - 3 cups
Turmeric - 1-inch
Lemon - 1

PROCEDURE

All ingredients should be thoroughly washed and dry before juicing.
Run each product through the juicer one at a time until all of them are juiced.
Serve right away with ice or without ice.

NUTRITION PER SERVING:

Calories: 187 | fat 1.1g | carbs 34.4g | protein 12.1g | sugar 13g

14.6 Blub Juice

Prep Time: 5 minutes | Cook Time: 0 minutes | Servings: 4

INGREDIENTS

Blueberries - 1 cup
Peaches - 5
Chard - 1 cup

PROCEDURE

All ingredients should be thoroughly washed and dry before juicing.
Run each product through the juicer one at a time until all of them are juiced.
Serve right away with ice or without ice.

NUTRITION PER SERVING:

Calories: 96 | fat 0.7g | carbs 23.1g | protein 2.2g | sugar 21.2g

14.7 Currant Juice

Prep Time: 5 minutes | Cook Time: 0 minutes | Servings: 1

INGREDIENTS

Raspberries - 1 cup
Black currants - ½ cup

PROCEDURE

All ingredients should be thoroughly washed and dry before juicing.
Run each product through the juicer one at a time until all of them are juiced.
Serve right away with ice or without ice.

NUTRITION PER SERVING:

Calories: 352 | fat 24g | carbs 41.1g | protein 2.3g | sugar 27.1g

14.8 Cor Juice

Prep Time: 2 minutes | Cook Time: 0 minutes | Servings: 2

INGREDIENTS
coriander - ½ bunch
green apples - 2
celery stalks - 1
grapes 1- cup

PROCEDURE
All ingredients should be thoroughly washed and dry before juicing.
Run each product through the juicer one at a time until all of them are juiced.
Serve right away with ice or without ice.

NUTRITION PER SERVING:
Calories: 149 | fat 0.6g | carbs 39.1g | protein 1g | sugar 30.8g

14.9 Rib Juice

Prep Time: 5 minutes | Cook Time: 0 minutes | Servings: 2

INGREDIENTS
ribs celery - 3
beet - ½
blueberries - 1 cup

PROCEDURE
All ingredients should be thoroughly washed and dry before juicing.
Run each product through the juicer one at a time until all of them are juiced.
Serve right away with ice or without ice.

NUTRITION PER SERVING:
Calories: 56 | fat 0.3g | carbs 13.6g | protein 1.1g | sugar 9.5g

14.10 Achler Juice

Prep Time: 5 minutes | Cook Time: 0 minutes | Servings: 2

Ingredients
ribs celery - 2
carrot - 1
spinach - 2 cups
lime - 1

PROCEDURE
All ingredients should be thoroughly washed and dry before juicing.
Run each product through the juicer one at a time until all of them are juiced.
Serve right away with ice or without ice.

NUTRITION PER SERVING:
Calories: 30 | fat 0.2g | carbs 6.9g | protein 1.5g | sugar 2.4g

14.11 Pars Juice

Prep Time: 5 minutes | Cook Time: 0 minutes | Servings: 2

INGREDIENTS
ribs celery - 2
carrot - 1
parsley - 1 cup
cucumber - 1 cup

PROCEDURE
All ingredients should be thoroughly washed and dry before juicing.
Run each product through the juicer one at a time until all of them are juiced.
Serve right away with ice or without ice.

NUTRITION PER SERVING:
Calories: 41 | fat 0.4g | carbs 8.7g | protein 1.9g | sugar 3.5g

14.12 Carrer Juice

Prep Time: 5 minutes | Cook Time: 0 minutes | Servings: 2

INGREDIENTS

beet - 1
apple - 1
carrot - 1
turmeric - 1-inch
ginger - 1-inch

PROCEDURE

All ingredients should be thoroughly washed and dry before juicing.
Run each product through the juicer one at a time until all of them are juiced.
Serve right away with ice or without ice.

NUTRITION PER SERVING:

Calories: 145 | fat 1.5g | carbs 33.6g | protein 2.7g | sugar 17.6g

14.13 Flower Juice

Prep Time: 10 minutes | Cook Time: 0 minutes | Servings: 2

INGREDIENTS

broccoli - ½ cup
cauliflower - ½ cup
apple - 1
courgette - ½
lemon - 1

PROCEDURE

All ingredients should be thoroughly washed and dry before juicing.
Run each product through the juicer one at a time until all of them are juiced.
Serve right away with ice or without ice.

NUTRITION PER SERVING:

Calories: 87 | fat 0.5g | carbs 22.1g | protein 2.3g | sugar 14g

14.14 Ava Juice

Prep Time: 5 minutes | Cook Time: 0 minutes | Servings: 3

INGREDIENTS

Apple - 2
carrots - 2
Avocado - 1
Blueberries - 1 cup

PROCEDURE

All ingredients should be thoroughly washed and dry before juicing.
Run each product through the juicer one at a time until all of them are juiced.
Serve right away with ice or without ice.

NUTRITION PER SERVING:

Calories: 258 | fat 13.5g | carbs 37.3g | protein 2.4g | sugar 22.6g

14.15 Grant Juice

Prep Time: 10 minutes | Cook Time: 0 minutes | Servings: 2

INGREDIENTS

Pomegranate seeds - 1 cup
Orange - ½
Broccoli - 1/3
Green Apple - 1

PROCEDURE

All ingredients should be thoroughly washed and dry before juicing.
Run each product through the juicer one at a time until all of them are juiced.
Serve right away with ice or without ice.

NUTRITION PER SERVING:

Calories: 169 | fat 3g | carbs 42.1g | protein 2g | sugar 26.3g

15 Weight Loss Juices

These juices are created to help people lose weight by allowing them to eat less solid food while still getting enough nutrients from the juice. These juices are generally low in Calories: and high in fibre, making them perfect for weight loss.

15.1 Blue Range Juice

Prep Time: 5 minutes | Cook Time: 0 minutes | Servings: 1

INGREDIENTS
blueberries - 1 cup
oranges - 2
pink grapefruit - 1

PROCEDURE
All ingredients should be thoroughly washed and dry before juicing.
Run each product through the juicer one at a time until all of them are juiced.
Serve right away with ice or without ice.

NUTRITION PER SERVING:
Calories: 238 | fat 1g | carbs 60g | protein 4g | sugar 46g

15.2 Pink Pop Juice

Prep Time: 5 minutes | Cook Time: 0 minutes | Servings: 1

INGREDIENTS
watermelon - 2 cups
orange - 1

PROCEDURE
All ingredients should be thoroughly washed and dry before juicing.
Run each product through the juicer one at a time until all of them are juiced.
Serve right away with ice or without ice.

NUTRITION PER SERVING:
Calories: 136 | fat 0.6g | carbs 34g | protein 2.7g | sugar 27g

15.3 Weet Juice

Prep Time: 5 minutes | Cook Time: 0 minutes | Servings: 1

INGREDIENTS
sweet potato, peeled - 1
stalks celery - 4
spinach - ½ cup
zucchini - 1
cucumber - 1

PROCEDURE
All ingredients should be thoroughly washed and dry before juicing.
Run each product through the juicer one at a time until all of them are juiced.
Serve right away with ice or without ice.

NUTRITION PER SERVING:
Calories: 219 | fat 1.4g | carbs 48g | protein 8g | sugar 18g

15.4 Fritcu Juice

Prep Time: 15 minutes | Cook Time: 0 minutes | Servings: 2

INGREDIENTS
beet - 1
carrots - 5
stalks celery - 2
cucumber - 1
grapefruit - 1
kiwi - 1
plum - 1
pears - 2
apples - 2

PROCEDURE

All ingredients should be thoroughly washed and dry before juicing.
Run each product through the juicer one at a time until all of them are juiced.
Serve right away with ice or without ice.

NUTRITION PER SERVING:

Calories: 606 | fat 2.4g | carbs 152g | protein 10g | sugar 94g

15.5   Pell Juice

Prep Time: 5 minutes | Cook Time: 0 minutes | Servings: 1

INGREDIENTS

apples - 2
watermelon - 3 cups

PROCEDURE

All ingredients should be thoroughly washed and dry before juicing.
Run each product through the juicer one at a time until all of them are juiced.
Serve right away with ice or without ice.

NUTRITION PER SERVING:

Calories: 242 | fat 1g | carbs 62g | protein 3.4g | sugar 50g

15.6   Tom Juice

Prep Time: minutes | Cook Time: 0 minutes | Servings: 4

INGREDIENTS

tomatoes - 2
stalks celery - 2
radishes - 3-4
red bell pepper - 1
yellow banana pepper - 1
fresh jalapeño pepper - 1

green onions, seeded - 3

PROCEDURE

All ingredients should be thoroughly washed and dry before juicing.
Run each product through the juicer one at a time until all of them are juiced.
Serve right away with ice or without ice.

NUTRITION PER SERVING:

Calories: 40 | fat 0g | carbs 9g | protein 1.7g | sugar 3.7g

15.7   Peman Juice

Prep Time: 5 minutes | Cook Time: 0 minutes | Servings: 1

INGREDIENTS

pears - 2
mango - 1
spinach - 1 cup

PROCEDURE

All ingredients should be thoroughly washed and dry before juicing.
Run each product through the juicer one at a time until all of them are juiced.
Serve right away with ice or without ice.

NUTRITION PER SERVING:

Calories: 33 | fat 1g | carbs 9g | protein 1g | sugar 6g

15.8   Mont Juice

Prep Time: 5 minutes | Cook Time: 0 minutes | Servings: 2

INGREDIENTS

beets - 2
carrots - 3
lemon - 1
apple - 1

kale leaves - 5
stalks celery - 4
ginger - 1-inch

PROCEDURE

All ingredients should be thoroughly washed and
dry before juicing
Run each product through the juicer one at a time
until all of them are juiced.
Serve right away with ice or without ice.

NUTRITION PER SERVING:

Calories: 135 | fat 1g | carbs 38g | protein 6g |
sugar 20g

15.9 Gerg Juice

Prep Time: 10 minutes | Cook Time: 0 minutes |
Servings: 1

Ingredients
pineapple - 1/3 cup
watermelon - 2 slices
ginger - 1-inch
lemon - 1
mint leaves - handful

PROCEDURE

All ingredients should be thoroughly washed and
dry before juicing.
Run each product through the juicer one at a time
until all of them are juiced.
Serve right away with ice or without ice.

NUTRITION PER SERVING:

Calories: 265 | fat 1.9g | carbs 65.3g | protein g5.6
| sugar 42.3g

15.10 Bloodli Juice

Prep Time: 5 minutes | Cook Time: 0 minutes |
Servings: 3

INGREDIENTS

Blood Oranges - 6
Serrano Chili - 2

PROCEDURE

All ingredients should be thoroughly washed and
dry before juicing.
Run each product through the juicer one at a time
until all of them are juiced.
Serve right away with ice or without ice.

NUTRITION PER SERVING:

Calories: 180 | fat 0.8g | carbs 43.7g | protein 4g |
sugar 34.5g

15.11 Sumber Juice

Prep Time: 10 minutes | Cook Time: 0 minutes |
Servings: 3

INGREDIENTS

cucumbers - 2
celery stalks - 4
red apples - 2
kale - 3 bunches
lemon - 1
spinach - 1 handful

PROCEDURE

All ingredients should be thoroughly washed and
dry before juicing.
Run each product through the juicer one at a time
until all of them are juiced.
Serve right away with ice or without ice.

NUTRITION PER SERVING:

Calories: 151 | fat 0.6g | carbs 37.3g | protein 4.3g
| sugar 19.6g

15.12 Cabler Juice

Prep Time: 5 minutes | Cook Time: 0 minutes |
Servings: 2

INGREDIENTS

purple cabbage leaves - 3-4
sticks of celery - 2
pears - 2

ginger root - 1-inch

PROCEDURE

All ingredients should be thoroughly washed and dry before juicing.
Run each product through the juicer one at a time until all of them are juiced.
Serve right away with ice or without ice.

NUTRITION PER SERVING:

Calories: 138 | fat 0.5g | carbs 35.2g | protein 1.4g | sugar 21.8g

15.13 Ramith Juice

Prep Time: 10 minutes | Cook Time: 0 minutes | Servings: 1

INGREDIENTS

beets - ½
Granny Smith apples -1
carrots - ½
cucumber - ½
ginger - 2-inch

PROCEDURE

All ingredients should be thoroughly washed and dry before juicing.
Run each product through the juicer one at a time until all of them are juiced.
Serve right away with ice or without ice.

NUTRITION PER SERVING:

Calories: 277 | fat 2.5g | carbs 65.5g | protein 5.4g | sugar 32.2g

15.14 Sleaf Juice

Prep Time: 5 minutes | Cook Time: 0 minutes | Servings: 1

INGREDIENTS

parsley - ½ cup

Ginger - ½ -inch
Cucumber - 1
lemon - 1
Apple - 1

PROCEDURE

All ingredients should be thoroughly washed and dry before juicing.
Run each product through the juicer one at a time until all of them are juiced.
Serve right away with ice or without ice.

NUTRITION PER SERVING:

Calories: 210 | fat 1.5g | carbs 53.1g | protein 4.6g | sugar 29.9g

15.15 Parpin Juice

Prep Time: 10 minutes | Cook Time: 0 minutes | Servings: 3

INGREDIENTS

ginger - ½ inch
cucumber - 1
kale - ½ bunch
parsley - ¼ cup
celery stalks - 2
pineapple - ½ cup
lemon - ¼
beet - 1
apple - 1

PROCEDURE

All ingredients should be thoroughly washed and dry before juicing.
Run each product through the juicer one at a time until all of them are juiced.
Serve right away with ice or without ice.

NUTRITION PER SERVING:

Calories: 105 | fat g0.1 | carbs 25.6g | protein 2.6g | sugar 15.5g

16 Detoxifying and Cleansing Juices

Detoxification is a long-term process that necessitates lifestyle and dietary adjustments. Cleansing is a short-term diet that aims to rid the body of toxins and cleanse the digestive tract. These juices provide therapeutic nourishment while also eliminating toxins and waste from the body.

16.1 Clime Juice

Prep Time: 5 minutes | Cook Time: 0 minutes | Servings: 2

INGREDIENTS
stalks celery - 2
cucumber - ½
lime - ½
cilantro - 1 cup
kale - 1 cup
green apple - 1

PROCEDURE
All ingredients should be thoroughly washed and dry before juicing.
Run each product through the juicer one at a time until all of them are juiced.
Serve right away with ice or without ice.

NUTRITION PER SERVING:
Calories: 93 | fat 0g | carbs 23.2g | protein 2.1g | sugar 13.3g

16.2 Inler Juice

Prep Time: 10 minutes | Cook Time: 0 minutes | Servings: 3

INGREDIENTS
stalks celery - 2
cucumber - ½
1 ginger - 1-inch
parsley - ½ cup
lemon - ½
green apple - 1
spinach - 2 cups

PROCEDURE
All ingredients should be thoroughly washed and dry before juicing.
Run each product through the juicer one at a time until all of them are juiced.
Serve right away with ice or without ice.

Nutrition per serving:
Calories: 76 | fat 0.7g | carbs 18g | protein 2g | sugar 9.2g

16.3 Celet Juice

Prep Time: 5 minutes | Cook Time: 0 minutes | Servings: 4

INGREDIENTS
ginger - 1-inch
beets - 3
carrots - 3
stalks celery - 3

PROCEDURE
All ingredients should be thoroughly washed and dry before juicing.
Run each product through the juicer one at a time until all of them are juiced.
Serve right away with ice or without ice.

NUTRITION PER SERVING:
Calories: 89 | fat 0.5g | carbs 20g | protein 2.8g | sugar 11.4g

16.4 Pime Juice

Prep Time: 10 minutes | Cook Time: 0 minutes | Servings: 4

INGREDIENTS

stalks kale - 3
spinach - 1 cup
pear - 1
lime - ½
stalks celery - 3
cucumber - ½

PROCEDURE

All ingredients should be thoroughly washed and dry before juicing.
Run each product through the juicer one at a time until all of them are juiced.
Serve right away with ice or without ice.

NUTRITION PER SERVING:

Calories: 34 | fat 0.2g | carbs 8.5g | protein 0.9g | sugar 4.3g

16.5 Ginery Juice

Prep Time: 5 minutes | Cook Time: 0 minutes | Servings: 4

INGREDIENTS

carrots - 4
ginger - 1-inch
orange - 1
lemon - ½
stalks celery - 3

PROCEDURE

All ingredients should be thoroughly washed and dry before juicing.
Run each product through the juicer one at a time until all of them are juiced.
Serve right away with ice or without ice.

NUTRITION PER SERVING:

Calories: 63 | fat 0.3g | carbs 15g | protein 1.4g | sugar 7.7g

16.6 Pimber Juice

Prep Time: 5 minutes | Cook Time: 0 minutes | Servings: 3

INGREDIENTS

cucumber - 1
parsley - 1 cup
spinach - 1 cup
green apples - 2

PROCEDURE

All ingredients should be thoroughly washed and dry before juicing.
Run each product through the juicer one at a time until all of them are juiced.
Serve right away with ice or without ice.

NUTRITION PER SERVING:

Calories: 102 | fat 0.6g | carbs 25.8g | protein 1.9g | sugar 17.4g

16.7 Stan Juice

Prep Time: 5 minutes | Cook Time: 0 minutes | Servings: 3

INGREDIENTS

pineapple - 1 cup
lemon - ½
carrots - 2
stalks celery - 2
ginger - 1 cm

PROCEDURE

All ingredients should be thoroughly washed and dry before juicing.
Run each product through the juicer one at a time until all of them are juiced.
Serve right away with ice or without ice.

NUTRITION PER SERVING:

Calories: 77 | fat 0.6g | carbs 18.1g | protein 1.6g | sugar 8g

16.8 Minch Juice

Prep Time: 5 minutes | Cook Time: 0 minutes | Servings: 3

INGREDIENTS

stalks celery - 2
cucumber - ½
spinach - 2 cups
mint leaves - 3 cups
pineapple -1 cup
lemon - ½

PROCEDURE

All ingredients should be thoroughly washed and dry before juicing.

Run each product through the juicer one at a time until all of them are juiced.

Serve right away with ice or without ice.

NUTRITION PER SERVING:

Calories: 82 | fat 0.9g | carbs 17.8g | protein 4.3g | sugar 6.5g

16.9 Graner Juice

Prep Time: 5 minutes | Cook Time: 0 minutes | Servings: 3

INGREDIENTS

carrots - 4
ginger - 1-inch
green apple - 2

PROCEDURE

All ingredients should be thoroughly washed and dry before juicing.

Run each product through the juicer one at a time until all of them are juiced.

Serve right away with ice or without ice.

NUTRITION PER SERVING:

Calories: 128 | fat 0.6g | carbs 32.1g | protein 1.5g | sugar 19.6g

16.10 Celmon Juice

Prep Time: 5 minutes | Cook Time: 0 minutes | Servings: 4

INGREDIENTS

beet - 1
carrots - 2
stalks celery - 3
lemon - ½
ginger - 1-inch
green apple - 1

PROCEDURE

All ingredients should be thoroughly washed and dry before juicing.

Run each product through the juicer one at a time until all of them are juiced.

Serve right away with ice or without ice.

NUTRITION PER SERVING:

Calories: 69 | fat 0.4g | carbs 16.7g | protein 1.3g | sugar 9.7g

16.11 Romer Juice

Prep Time: 10 minutes | Cook Time: 0 minutes | Servings: 3

INGREDIENTS

cucumber - ½
stalks celery - 2
romaine lettuce - 1 cup
broccoli - 1 cup
green apple - 2
lime - ½

PROCEDURE

All ingredients should be thoroughly washed and dry before juicing.

Run each product through the juicer one at a time until all of them are juiced.

Serve right away with ice or without ice.

NUTRITION PER SERVING:

Calories: 101 | fat 0.5g | carbs 25.6g | protein 1.8g | sugar 17.2g

16.12 Let Green Juice

Prep Time: 5 minutes | Cook Time: 0 minutes | Servings: 3

INGREDIENTS

lettuce   1 cup

cucumber - 1

stalks celery - 4

green apple - 1

lemon - 1

PROCEDURE

All ingredients should be thoroughly washed and dry before juicing.

Run each product through the juicer one at a time until all of them are juiced.

Serve right away with ice or without ice.

Nutrition per serving:

Calories: 64 | fat 0.4g | carbs 16.6g | protein 1.3g | sugar g

10.3

16.13 Cilaner Juice

Prep Time: 10 minutes | Cook Time: 0 minutes | Servings: 3

INGREDIENTS

cucumbers - 2

parsley - handful

cilantro - handful

leaves kale - 2

Swiss chard – 4 leaves

stalks celery - 2

ginger peeled - 1-inch

lemons - 2

PROCEDURE

All ingredients should be thoroughly washed and dry before juicing.

Run each product through the juicer one at a time until all of them are juiced.

Serve right away with ice or without ice.

NUTRITION PER SERVING:

Calories: 79 | fat 0.7g | carbs 18.3g | protein 4.2g | sugar 5.3g

16.14 Kaler Juice

Prep Time: 5 minutes | Cook Time: 0 minutes | Servings: 2

INGREDIENTS

beet - 1

cucumber - 1

stalks celery - 4

leaves kale - 4

lemon - 1

PROCEDURE

All ingredients should be thoroughly washed and dry before juicing.

Run each product through the juicer one at a time until all of them are juiced.

Serve right away with ice or without ice.

NUTRITION PER SERVING:

Calories: 65 | fat 0.4g | carbs 15.4g | protein 2.8g | sugar 7.6g

16.15 Poter Juice

Prep Time: 5 minutes | Cook Time: 0 minutes | Servings: 2

INGREDIENTS

sweet potatoes - 2

carrots - 2

ginger - 1-inch

PROCEDURE

All ingredients should be thoroughly washed and dry before juicing.

Run each product through the juicer one at a time until all of them are juiced.

Serve right away with ice or without ice.

NUTRITION PER SERVING:

Calories: 204 | fat 0.7g | carbs 47.6g | protein 3.2g | sugar 3.9g

17 Immune Boosting Juices

These fresh Immune Boosting Juice will help to strengthen your immune system. It's a combination of different fruits, vegetables, and herbs. These juices are high in vitamins, which might assist your immune system. These refreshing juices are appealing due to the natural sweetness of the fruits. It's the ideal technique to give oneself a competitive advantage.

17.1 Meric juice

Prep Time: 5 minutes | Cook Time: 0 minutes | Servings: 1

INGREDIENTS

mint - ½ cup
apple - 1
fresh turmeric - 1-inch
ginger - 1-inch
lemon - 1

PROCEDURE

All ingredients should be thoroughly washed and dry before juicing.
Run each product through the juicer one at a time until all of them are juiced.
Serve right away with ice or without ice.

NUTRITION PER SERVING:

Calories: 253 | fat g3.2 | carbs 58g | protein 3.9g | sugar 25.2g

17.2 Parle Juice

Prep Time: 5 minutes | Cook Time: 0 minutes | Servings: 2

INGREDIENTS

apple - 1
stalks celery - 4
bunch parsley - 1 bunch

PROCEDURE

All ingredients should be thoroughly washed and dry before juicing.

Run each product through the juicer one at a time until all of them are juiced.
Serve right away with ice or without ice.

Nutrition per serving:
Calories: 74 | fat 0.5g | carbs 18.3g | protein 1.4g | sugar 12.3g

17.3 Ranrot Juice

Prep Time: 5 minutes | Cook Time: 0 minutes | Servings: 2

INGREDIENTS

carrots - 2
parsley - ½ cup
oranges - 2

PROCEDURE

All ingredients should be thoroughly washed and dry before juicing.
Run each product through the juicer one at a time until all of them are juiced.
Serve right away with ice or without ice.

NUTRITION PER SERVING:

Calories: 117 | fat 0.3g | carbs 28.6g | protein 2.7g | sugar 20.3g

17.4 Plumb Juice

Prep Time: 5 minutes | Cook Time: 0 minutes | Servings: 2

INGREDIENTS

beets - 2
purple cabbage - ¼
plums - 4

PROCEDURE

All ingredients should be thoroughly washed and dry before juicing.

Run each product through the juicer one at a time until all of them are juiced.

Serve right away with ice or without ice.

NUTRITION PER SERVING:

Calories: 106 | fat 0.6g | carbs 26.5g | protein 2.8g | sugar 22.2g

17.5   Pale Juice

Prep Time: 5 minutes | Cook Time: 0 minutes | Servings: 1

INGREDIENTS

kale - 1 bunch

cucumber - 1

pear - 1

PROCEDURE

All ingredients should be thoroughly washed and dry before juicing.

Run each product through the juicer one at a time until all of them are juiced.

Serve right away with ice or without ice.

NUTRITION PER SERVING:

Calories: 159 | fat 0.5g | carbs 39.1g | protein 4.5g | sugar 18.6g

17.6   Turo Juice

Prep Time: 5 minutes | Cook Time: 0 minutes | Servings: 2

INGREDIENTS

Carrot - 1

Apple - 1

Ginger - 1-inch

Turmeric - 1-inch

Orange - 2

PROCEDURE

All ingredients should be thoroughly washed and dry before juicing.

Run each product through the juicer one at a time until all of them are juiced.

Serve right away with ice or without ice.

NUTRITION PER SERVING:

Calories: 210 | fat 1.6g | carbs 50.2g | protein 3.6g | sugar 30.8g

17.7   Genmon Juice

Prep Time: 10 minutes | Cook Time: 0 minutes | Servings: 2

INGREDIENTS

Lettuce leaves - 2

Cucumber - ½

Parsley - ½ cup

Spinach - ½ cup

Green apples - 2

Lemon - ½

Ginger - 1-inch

PROCEDURE

All ingredients should be thoroughly washed and dry before juicing.

Run each product through the juicer one at a time until all of them are juiced.

Serve right away with ice or without ice.

NUTRITION PER SERVING:

Calories: 164 | fat 1.1g | carbs 41.2g | protein g2.6 | sugar 25.2g

17.8   Carlt Juice

Prep Time: 5 minutes | Cook Time: 0 minutes | Servings: 2

INGREDIENTS

Beet - ½

carrot - ½

Lemon - ½

Apple - 1

Celery stalk - 1

Kale - handful

Ginger - 1-inch

PROCEDURE

All ingredients should be thoroughly washed and dry before juicing.

Run each product through the juicer one at a time until all of them are juiced.

Serve right away with ice or without ice.

NUTRITION PER SERVING:

Calories: 122 | fat 0.7g | carbs 29.5g | protein 2.7g | sugar 15g

17.9 Tomta Juice

Prep Time: 5 minutes | Cook Time: 0 minutes | Servings: 2

INGREDIENTS

Kale - ½ cup
Parsley - ½ cup
Celery Stalk - 1
Tomato - 1
Lemon - ½
Pears - 2

PROCEDURE

All ingredients should be thoroughly washed and dry before juicing.

Run each product through the juicer one at a time until all of them are juiced.

Serve right away with ice or without ice.

NUTRITION PER SERVING:

Calories: 145 | fat 0.5g | carbs 37g | protein 2.2g | sugar 21.7g

17.10 Peener Juice

Prep Time: minutes | Cook Time: 0 minutes | Servings: 2

INGREDIENTS

Celery Stalks - 2
Spinach - ½ cup
Green Apple - 1
Cucumber - 1

PROCEDURE

All ingredients should be thoroughly washed and dry before juicing.

Run each product through the juicer one at a time until all of them are juiced.

Serve right away with ice or without ice.

NUTRITION PER SERVING:

Calories: 85 | fat 0.4g | carbs 21.6g | protein 1.6g | sugar 14.4g

17.11 Mater Juice

Prep Time: 5 minutes | Cook Time: 0 minutes | Servings: 2

INGREDIENTS

Beet - 1
Carrot - 1
Tomato - 1
Cucumber - 1
Mint Leaves - 3
Ginger - 1-inch
Lime - ½

PROCEDURE

All ingredients should be thoroughly washed and dry before juicing.

Run each product through the juicer one at a time until all of them are juiced.

Serve right away with ice or without ice.

NUTRITION PER SERVING:

Calories: 93 | fat 0.8g | carbs 21g | protein 3.3g | sugar 9.1g

17.12 Berint Juice

Prep Time: 5 minutes | Cook Time: 0 minutes | Servings: 2

Ingredients
Blueberry - ½ cup
Raspberry - ½ cup
Blackberry - ½ cup
Mint leaves - 3

PROCEDURE

All ingredients should be thoroughly washed and dry before juicing.

Run each product through the juicer one at a time until all of them are juiced.

Serve right away with ice or without ice.

NUTRITION PER SERVING:

Calories: 55 | fat 0.6g | carbs 12.9g | protein 1.3g | sugar 6.7g

17.13 Orim Juice

Prep Time: 5 minutes | Cook Time: 0 minutes | Servings: 2

INGREDIENTS

Oranges - 2
Lemon - ½
Lime - ½
Pineapple - 1 slice
Ginger - 1 oz
Turmeric - 1 oz

PROCEDURE

All ingredients should be thoroughly washed and dry before juicing.

Run each product through the juicer one at a time until all of them are juiced.

Serve right away with ice or without ice.

NUTRITION PER SERVING:

Calories: 154 | fat 1.5g | carbs 36.1g | protein 3.3g | sugar 20.1g

17.14 Stiwi Juice

Prep Time: 5 minutes | Cook Time: 0 minutes | Servings: 2

INGREDIENTS

Strawberries - 2 cups
Kiwi 1 - cup

PROCEDURE

All ingredients should be thoroughly washed and dry before juicing.

Run each product through the juicer one at a time until all of them are juiced.

Serve right away with ice or without ice.

NUTRITION PER SERVING:

Calories: 100 | fat 0.9g | carbs 24g | protein 2g | sugar 15g

17.15 Parran Juice

Prep Time: 10 minutes | Cook Time: 0 minutes | Servings: 2

INGREDIENTS

Apple - 1
Celery - 1
Parsley - ½ cup
Carrot - 1
Orange - 1
Ginger - 1-inch
Lemon - 1

PROCEDURE

All ingredients should be thoroughly washed and dry before juicing.

Run each product through the juicer one at a time until all of them are juiced.

Serve right away with ice or without ice.

NUTRITION PER SERVING:

Calories: 154 | fat 1g | carbs 38g | protein 2.9g | sugar 22.9g

18 Anti-Aging and energizing juices

These juices are high in antioxidants, chlorogenic acids, and pectin, making them great anti-aging juices. Drinking these juices on a regular basis helps to reduce fine lines and wrinkles, as well as acts as an antibacterial to protect your brain from the detrimental effects of aging and enhance physical endurance, making you feel more energized throughout the day.

18.1 Cucar Juice

Prep Time: 5 minutes | Cook Time: 0 minutes | Servings: 1

INGREDIENTS
Cucumber - ¼
Carrot juice - ¼ cup
Apple
Kale

PROCEDURE
All ingredients should be thoroughly washed and dry before juicing.
Run each product through the juicer one at a time until all of them are juiced.
Serve right away with ice or without ice.

NUTRITION PER SERVING:
Calories: 142 | fat 0.5g | carbs 36.8g | protein 1.7g | sugar 25.2g

18.2 Reet Juice

Prep Time: minutes | Cook Time: 0 minutes | Servings: 1

INGREDIENTS
yellow Beetroot - ½
Lettuce leaves - 5
apple - 1
Lemon - 1
ginger - 1-inch

PROCEDURE
All ingredients should be thoroughly washed and dry before juicing.
Run each product through the juicer one at a time until all of them are juiced.

Serve right away with ice or without ice.

NUTRITION PER SERVING:
Calories: 206 | fat 1.6g | carbs 51.1g | protein 3.4g | sugar 29g

18.3 Pully Juice

Prep Time: 5 minutes | Cook Time: 0 minutes | Servings: 1

INGREDIENTS
Blueberries - 1 cup
Apple - 1

PROCEDURE
All ingredients should be thoroughly washed and dry before juicing.
Run each product through the juicer one at a time until all of them are juiced.
Serve right away with ice or without ice.

NUTRITION PER SERVING:
Calories: 199 | fat 0.9g | carbs 51.8g | protein 1.7g | sugar 37.6g

18.4 Talker Juice

Prep Time: 5 minutes | Cook Time: 0 minutes | Servings: 3

INGREDIENTS
Cucumber - 1
Carrots - 2
grapes - ½ cup
Apples - 2
Celery stalk - 1

PROCEDURE

All ingredients should be thoroughly washed and dry before juicing.

Run each product through the juicer one at a time until all of them are juiced.

Serve right away with ice or without ice.

NUTRITION PER SERVING:

Calories: 120 | fat 0.4g | carbs 31g | protein 1.5g | sugar 21.7g

18.5 Chunker Juice

Prep Time: minutes | Cook Time: 0 minutes | Servings: 1

INGREDIENTS

watermelon chunks - 1 cup

Strawberries - ½ cup

lime juice - ¼

ginger - 1-inch

PROCEDURE

All ingredients should be thoroughly washed and dry before juicing.

Run each product through the juicer one at a time until all of them are juiced.

Serve right away with ice or without ice.

NUTRITION PER SERVING:

Calories: 148 | fat 1.4g | carbs 34.4g | protein 3.3g | sugar 18.6g

18.6 Ranith juice

Prep Time: 5 minutes | Cook Time: 0 minutes | Servings: 4

INGREDIENTS

kale - 1 bunch

celery stalks - 6

lemon - 2

ginger - 2-inch

cucumber - 2

granny smith apple - 1

PROCEDURE

All ingredients should be thoroughly washed and dry before juicing.

Run each product through the juicer one at a time until all of them are juiced.

Serve right away with ice or without ice.

NUTRITION PER SERVING:

Calories: 67 | fat 1g | carbs 16g | protein 2g | sugar 8g

18.7 Darin Juice

Prep Time: 5 minutes | Cook Time: 0 minutes | Servings: 3

INGREDIENTS

Mandarins - 10

Oranges - 5

Grapefruit - 1

Lemon - ½

Lime - ¼

PROCEDURE

All ingredients should be thoroughly washed and dry before juicing.

Run each product through the juicer one at a time until all of them are juiced.

Serve right away with ice or without ice.

NUTRITION PER SERVING:

Calories: 259 | fat 0.5g | carbs 66g | protein 5g | sugar 59g

18.8 Celes Juice

Prep Time: 10 minutes | Cook Time: 0 minutes | Servings: 3

INGREDIENTS

Apples - 4

Celery stalks - 6

Kale Leaves - 2

PROCEDURE

All ingredients should be thoroughly washed and dry before juicing.

Run each product through the juicer one at a time until all of them are juiced.

Serve right away with ice or without ice.

NUTRITION PER SERVING:

Calories: 139 | fat 0.5g | carbs 36g | protein 1g | sugar 26g

18.9 Brob Juice

Prep Time: 5 minutes | Cook Time: 0 minutes | Servings: 1

INGREDIENTS

celery stalks - 2
cucumber - 1
green apple - ½
broccoli head - ½
fennel bulb - 1 whole

PROCEDURE

All ingredients should be thoroughly washed and dry before juicing.

Run each product through the juicer one at a time until all of them are juiced.

Serve right away with ice or without ice.

NUTRITION PER SERVING:

Calories: 158 | fat 1g | carbs 38.1g | protein 5.2g | sugar 18.5g

18.10 Potman Juice

Prep Time: 5 minutes | Cook Time: 0 minutes | Servings: 2

INGREDIENTS

sweet potato - ½
green apple - 1
mandarins - 4
lemon - ½

PROCEDURE

All ingredients should be thoroughly washed and dry before juicing.

Run each product through the juicer one at a time until all of them are juiced.

Serve right away with ice or without ice.

NUTRITION PER SERVING:

Calories: 161 | fat g0.7 | carbs 40.9g | protein 2.1g | sugar 28.5g

18.11 Pinles Juice

Prep Time: 5 minutes | Cook Time: 0 minutes | Servings: 3

INGREDIENTS

apples - 2
baby spinach - 3 cups
celery ribs - 2
cucumber - ½
lemon - ½
ginger - ½ -inch

PROCEDURE

All ingredients should be thoroughly washed and dry before juicing.

Run each product through the juicer one at a time until all of them are juiced.

Serve right away with ice or without ice.

NUTRITION PER SERVING:

Calories: 106 | fat 0.7g | carbs 26.5g | protein 2.1g | sugar 17.1g

18.12 Yelish Juice

Prep Time: 5 minutes | Cook Time: 0 minutes | Servings: 2

INGREDIENTS

yellow Beetroot - 1
Apple - 1
Celery stalks - 2

Carrots - 1-2
Lemon - ½
inch Ginger - ½ -inch

PROCEDURE

All ingredients should be thoroughly washed and dry before juicing.
Run each product through the juicer one at a time until all of them are juiced.
Serve right away with ice or without ice.

Nutrition per serving:
Calories: 123 | fat 0.6g | carbs 30.3g | protein 2.2g | sugar 19.2g

18.13 Cado Juice

Prep Time: 10 minutes | Cook Time: 0 minutes | Servings: 2

INGREDIENTS

green apples - 2
celery stalks - 2
cucumber - ½
spinach - 2 handfuls
lettuce leaves - 2
avocado - ½
banana - 1

PROCEDURE

All ingredients should be thoroughly washed and dry before juicing.
Run each product through the juicer one at a time until all of them are juiced.
Serve right away with ice or without ice.

NUTRITION PER SERVING:

Calories: 293 | fat 10.6g | carbs 53.1g | protein 3.7g | sugar 32.3g

18.14 Corang Juice

Prep Time: 5 minutes | Cook Time: 0 minutes | Servings: 1

INGREDIENTS

broccoli head - 1
oranges - 2
apple - 1

PROCEDURE

All ingredients should be thoroughly washed and dry before juicing.
Run each product through the juicer one at a time until all of them are juiced.
Serve right away with ice or without ice.

NUTRITION PER SERVING:

Calories: 369 | fat 1.6g | carbs 89.7g | protein 10.7g | sugar 61.6g

18.15 Canta Juice

Prep Time: 5 minutes | Cook Time: 0 minutes | Servings: 1

INGREDIENTS

cantaloupe - ½
carrots - 2
mango - 1

PROCEDURE

All ingredients should be thoroughly washed and dry before juicing.
Run each product through the juicer one at a time until all of them are juiced.
Serve right away with ice or without ice.

NUTRITION PER SERVING:

Calories: 275 | fat 1.4g | carbs 68g | protein 4.3g | sugar 57.3g

19 Frozen treats

These are the frozen treats containing the minerals, vitamins, and fibre to achieve your daily nutritional intakes and meet frozen sweet cravings without the restriction of having lots of carbs.

19.1 Iced Frappe

Prep Time: 5 minutes | Cook Time: 2 minutes | Servings: 2

INGREDIENTS

prepared Instant Espresso, completely cooled - ½ cup
ice cubes - 1 cup
milk - ¼ cup
sugar, or to taste - 2 tbsp.

PROCEDURE

Combine ice, cold espresso, milk, and sugar in a blender.
Begin blending on LOW and gradually raise the speed.
Blend for 30 seconds on high or until smooth.
Serve right away by dividing the frappe between two glasses.

NUTRITION FACTS: [PER SERVING]

Calories: 65 | fat 1g | carbs 13g | protein 0g | sugar 13g

19.2 Frappe Mocha

Prep Time: 5 minutes | Cook Time: 0 minutes | Servings: 2

INGREDIENTS

boiling water - ¼ cup
chocolate syrup - 4 ½ tsp.
crushed ice - ½ cup
fat-free milk - 1 cup
instant coffee - 1tsp.

Whipped topping and additional chocolate syrup, optional

PROCEDURE

Dissolve coffee in water in a bowl. Freeze the coffee mixture in an ice cube tray.
Combine the milk, chocolate syrup, and coffee ice cubes in a blender. Blend till smooth, covered. Blend in the crushed ice. Pour the blended mixture into chilled glasses and serve right away. If desired, top with whipped topping and more chocolate syrup.

NUTRITION FACTS: [PER SERVING]

Calories: 80 | fat 0g | carbs 15g | protein 5g | sugar 14g

19.3 Caramel Frappe

Prep Time: 5 minutes | Cook Time: 5 minutes | Servings: 2

INGREDIENTS

espresso coffee chilled - 3 tbsp.
milk - 1 ½ cup
sweetened condensed milk - ½ cup
caramel sauce - 2 tbsp.
ice - 2 cups
Whipped cream for garnish
More caramel sauce for garnish

PROCEDURE

Add all the caramel frappe ingredients into the blender; blend until completely smooth.
Fill a cup with caramel sauce; pour into it (to make it coffee house style).
Top the frappe with whipped cream; drizzle with caramel sauce before serving, if desired.

NUTRITION FACTS: [PER SERVING]

Calories: 408 | fat 13g | carbs 64g | protein 12g | sugar 51g

19.4 Lemon Italian Ice

Prep Time: 5 minutes | Cook Time: 5 minutes | Servings: 5

INGREDIENTS

water - 4 cups
granulated sugar - 1 cup
finely grated lemon zest - 1 tbsp.
freshly squeezed lemon juice - ¾ cup

PROCEDURE

In a medium saucepan add water, and boil over high heat. Add in the sugar and stir until constantly sugar is completely dissolved.
Bring water to a rolling boil.
Allow the water to cool before stirring in the lemon zest and juice.
Fill a baking pan halfway with the mixture and place it in the freezer.
Fill the baking pan halfway with the mixture.
Stir the crystals gently every 30 minutes or so, and leave until the mixture is smooth and all of the liquid has crystallized but not frozen solid—about 3 hours. As the mixture begins to freeze, you may need to scrape it with a fork.
Stir the stones gently.
To serve, scoop into tiny glasses.

NUTRITION FACTS: [PER SERVING]

Calories: 160 | fat 0.3g | carbs 41g | protein 0.3g | sugar 40.8g

19.5 Strawberry Italian Ice

Prep Time: 10 minutes | Cook Time: 0 minutes | Servings: 5

INGREDIENTS

apple juice, unsweetened - ¾ cup
lemon juice - 1-3 tbsp.
fresh strawberries, halved and hulled - 2 pints
Fresh mint, optional

PROCEDURE

In the blender, add apple juice, lemon juice, and strawberries; blend until smooth. Pour onto an 8-inch square steel dish that hasn't been greased. Cover the dish and freeze for approx. 2 to 3 hours, or until partially frozen.
Spoon into a mixing bowl and beat for 1-2 minutes on medium-low speed. Return to the dish and place in the freezer for 2-3 hours, or until stiff. Remove 10 minutes before serving from the freezer. If desired, garnish with mint.

NUTRITION FACTS: [PER SERVING]

Calories: 109 | fat 1g | carbs 27g | protein 1g | sugar g

19.6 Italian Ice

Prep Time: 60 minutes | Cook Time: 0 minutes | Servings: 4

INGREDIENTS

fresh lemon juice - 1 tbsp.
honey - 2 tbsp.
pineapple cubes - 3 cups
sugar - 2 tbsp.

PROCEDURE

In the food processor, add the fruit, sugar, honey, and lemon juice with 2 cups ice; process until chunky. Blend in 1 cup more ice until completely smooth.
Freeze for 30 minutes after pouring the mixture into a shallow baking dish. Scrape the ice mixture with a fork until it's mushy, after that freeze for another 2-3 hours or until stiff. Fill paper cups halfway with the mixture.

Nutrition facts: [per serving]
Calories: 117 | fat 0.2g | carbs 31g | protein 0.7g | sugar 26.9g

19.7 Pitcher Ice

Prep Time: 20 minutes | Cook Time: 0 minutes | Servings: 10

INGREDIENTS

raspberry syrup - 3 cups

lemon juice - ¾ cup
lemon, zested - 1
mint leaves, finely chopped - ¼ cup
crushed ice - 5 pounds

PROCEDURE

In a pitcher, combine the syrup, lemon juice, lemon zest, and mint. Refrigerate until ready to use.
In the food processor add ice; process until the ice is shaved.
In a serving dish, put 1 1/2 cups crushed ice. 3–4 teaspoons of the syrup mixture should be poured over the ice. Serve right away.

NUTRITION FACTS: [PER SERVING]
Calories: 235 | fat 0.2g | carbs 62.2g | protein 1.5g | sugar 58.1g

19.8 Fruit Sherbet

Prep Time: 5 minutes | Cook Time: 0 minutes | Servings: 4

INGREDIENTS
lemon juice - 1 cup
milk - 1 cup
orange juice - 1 cup
pineapple juice - ½ cup
sugar - 1 ½ cups

PROCEDURE
In the big pitcher, add lemon juice and sugar. Combine the orange juice, milk, and pineapple juice in a mixing bowl. Fill a plastic jar with the mixture and freeze until firm.

NUTRITION FACTS: [PER SERVING]
Calories 300 | fat 1.4g | carbs 95.6g | protein 2.8g | sugar 87.6g

19.9 Orange Sherbet

Prep Time: 15 minutes | Cook Time: 0 minutes | Servings: 4

INGREDIENTS
finely grated orange zest - 1 ½ tbsp.

kosher salt - ¼ tsp.
lemon juice, fresh - 1 tsp.
orange juice, fresh - 2 cups
sugar - ounces
vanilla extract - 1 tsp.
whole milk, cold - 1 ½ cups

PROCEDURE

In the food processor add all the sherbet ingredients, except the milk, and process for 1-2 minutes until the sugar is completely dissolved. In the large mixing bowl add the milk and sugar mixture and whisk to combine. Cover the bowl and chill for 1-2 hours or until the mixture reaches 40°F or lower.
Add the cooled sugar and milk mixture to an ice-cream machine halfway; process until it reaches soft-serve ice cream consistency. You may either serve right away or transfer to a lid container, freeze until stiff, about 3 hours.

NUTRITION FACTS: [PER SERVING]
Calories: 154 | fat 2g | carbs 34g | protein 2g | sugar 32g

19.10 Strawberry Sherbet

Prep Time: 5 minutes | Cook Time: 0 minutes | Servings: 2

INGREDIENTS
frozen strawberries - 1 cup
lemon juice - 1 tbsp.
kosher salt - 1 pinch
whole milk - ½ cup
ultrafine Baker's sugar, also called caster sugar - 1/3 cup

PROCEDURE
Freeze the strawberries (if using fresh strawberries), milk, and the food processor bowl and blade for at least 1 hour, or until the berries are solidly frozen. Add frozen strawberries, sugar, lemon juice, and salt into the food processor and pulse to roughly chop the berries. Then keep running the machine until it's almost smooth, but not quite.

Pour the cold milk down the feed tube into the strawberry combination while the machine is still working until the mixture is JUST mixed. Immediately spoon into dessert bowls and serve.

NUTRITION FACTS: [PER SERVING]

Calories: 190 | fat 2.3g | carbs 42.1g | protein 2.5g | sugar 39.9g

19.11 Cranberry Sherbet

Prep Time: 25 minutes | Cook Time: 20 minutes | Servings: 10

INGREDIENTS

2% milk - 1 cup
fresh or frozen cranberries - 4 cups
lemon juice - 1 tsp.
lemonade, frozen - 1 can (12 ounces)
orange juice, frozen - 1 can (12 ounces)
salt - ¼ tsp.
sugar - 2 ¾ cups
water - 4 cups

PROCEDURE

In a large saucepan. add cranberries and water; cook for 15 minutes over medium-low heat, or until the berries explode. Turn the heat off, add the sugar; stir until it is completely dissolved.
Fill a food processor halfway with the cranberry mixture. Cover and pulse the lemonade concentrate, orange juice concentrate, milk, lemon juice, and salt until smooth.
Fill the freezer ice cream cylinder two-thirds and freeze to the manufacturer's instructions. Keep the leftover sherbet mixture refrigerated until ready to freeze. Freeze for 4 hours or until stiff in a freezer.

NUTRITION FACTS: [PER SERVING]

Calories: 179 | fat 0g | carbs 45g | protein 1g | sugar 43g

19.12 Wild Popsicles

Prep Time: 4 minutes | Cook Time: 0 minutes | Servings: 4

INGREDIENTS

agave syrup - 1 tbsp.
cacao nibs - 1 tsp.
chopped pistachios - 2 tbsp.
coconut milk, full fat - ½ can
dried rose petals or buds - 1 tbsp.
wild strawberries - 2 cups

PROCEDURE

Strawberries should be washed and dried, and stems should be removed if necessary. Blend them together with the coconut milk and agave syrup in a blender for approx. 2-3 minutes, or until smooth. Pour the wild popsicle mixture into a popsicle mold, top with popsicle sticks, and set in the freezer for a few hours or overnight.
Remove the popsicles and the mold from the freezer once they've frozen. If the popsicles are stuck, run water over the mold and gently stir them around until they give up, and you can remove them.
Eat immediately after topping popsicles with chopped pistachios, rose petals, and chocolate nibs.

NUTRITION FACTS: [PER SERVING]

Calories: 183 | fat 14.83g | carbs 12.26g | protein 3.11g | sugar 6.6g

19.13 Green Popsicles

Prep Time: 10 minutes | Cook Time: 0 minutes | Servings: 8

INGREDIENTS

banana - 1
fresh spinach - 1 cup
grated fresh ginger - 1 tbsp.
honey - 2 tbsp.
kiwis - 2
milk - 1 cup
parsley - ¼ cup

PROCEDURE

Add milk, spinach, parsley, banana, 1 kiwi, honey, and ginger in the blender and blend until smooth, then taste and adjust the sweetness as needed.

The remaining kiwi should be peeled and sliced, with a piece or two going into each popsicle mold. Fill each mold halfway with a green smoothie, then freeze until firm (at least 6 hours).
To loosen the popsicles, remove them from the freezer and run them under warm water for a few seconds.

NUTRITION FACTS: [PER SERVING]
Calories: 45 | fat 1g | carbs 10g | protein 1g | sugar 7g

19.14 White Ice Pops

Prep Time: 10 minutes | Cook Time: 0 minutes | Servings: 10

INGREDIENTS
fresh blueberries - 1 cup
fresh raspberries - 1-1/2 cups
honey - 1-2 tbsp.
milk, divided - 1-3/4 cups 2%
vanilla extract - ¼ tsp.

PROCEDURE
Warm 1/4 cup milk in the microwave, then mix in honey until smooth. After that combine the remaining milk and the vanilla extract in a mixing bowl.
Fill molds halfway with berries and the remaining milk mixture. Holders for the top molds If you're using cups, place foil on top and poke the sticks through the foil. Freeze for approx. more than 30 minutes.

NUTRITION FACTS: [PER SERVING]
Calories: 51 | fat 2g | carbs 8g | protein 2g | sugar 6g

19.15 Avocado Ice Pops

Prep Time: 10 minutes | Cook Time: 0 minutes | Servings: 6

INGREDIENTS
chopped peeled avocado - 2 cups
grated lime rind - ½ tsp.
kosher salt - 1/8 tsp
lime juice - 2 tbsp.
sugar - 6 tbsp.
water - ¾ cup

PROCEDURE
Add water and sugar together in a medium saucepan. Cook for 4 minutes, often stirring to dissolve the sugar; set aside to cool. In the food processor, add sugar mixture, avocado, lime rind-juice, and kosher salt; process for approx.. 2-3 minutes or until smooth. Evenly distribute the ice pops mixture among 6 (4-ounce) ice-pop molds; cover with the lid. Freeze for at least 4-5 hours until completely frozen.

NUTRITION FACTS: [PER SERVING]
Calories: 130 | fat 7.3g | carbs g | protein g | sugar g

20 Conclusion

We have come to the end of our journey, but it's also the start of a new perspective on what fruits and vegetables can do for you. To help you get started, we've covered the basics and some of the benefits of power juicing in this book.

It is all about finding a balanced, healthy and making the greatest food choices we can on a daily basis. Adding juices is a terrific way to start experimenting with all the goodness nature offers. It doesn't have to be complicated or time-consuming. The most essential thing is to consume as much of these potent homemade juices as possible.

Do not hurry; take one step at a time, and one day at a time, and little changes like adding more fruits and vegetables to your diet will gradually lead to the healthier and more energized lifestyle you've been seeking. This isn't a diet. This is a long-term lifestyle modification. It's time to give your body a fresh start and take proper care of yourself. Never put off until tomorrow what you can do today. Today is your chance to shine and become a better version of yourself. Let's start our journey today with one of these juices.

21 Bibliography

Office of the Commissioner. (2021, June 15). *7 Tips for Cleaning Fruits, Vegetables*. U.S. Food and Drug Administration. Retrieved June 28, 2022, from https://www.fda.gov/consumers/consumer-updates/7-tips-cleaning-fruits-vegetables#:%7E:text=Gently%20rub%20product%20while%20holding,bacteria%20that%20may%20be%20present.

10 Reasons Why Juicing Can Improve Your Life. (n.d.). The Body Toolkit. Retrieved June 28, 2022, from https://www.thebodytoolkit.com/blog-article/10-reasons-why-juicing-can-improve-your-life

A. (2021, November 18). *Morning Green Juice*. The Petite Cook™. Retrieved June 28, 2022, from https://www.thepetitecook.com/morning-green-juice/

Fruits, Vegetables, Additives. (n.d.-a). Healthline. Retrieved June 28, 2022, from https://www.healthline.com/

Fruits, Vegetables, Additives. (n.d.-b). Medical News Today. Retrieved June 28, 2022, from https://www.medicalnewstoday.com/

Georgiou, C. R. N. (2017, March 10). *The Best Tips for Storing Your Juice*. Joe Cross. Retrieved June 28, 2022, from https://www.rebootwithjoe.com/the-best-tips-for-storing-your-juice/

Hill, R. A. D. (2020, April 24). *Does Green Juice Have Benefits? All You Need to Know*. Healthline. Retrieved June 28, 2022, from https://www.healthline.com/nutrition/green-juice-benefits

Jhawer, M. (2020, October 7). *Juices for Disease Prevention and Cure*. Medindia. Retrieved June 28, 2022, from https://www-medindia-net.cdn.ampproject.org/v/s/www.medindia.net/amp/patients/lifestyleandwellness/juices-for-detoxification-and-wellbeing-disease-prevention-and-cure.htm?amp_gsa=1&_js_v=a9&usqp=mq331AQKKAFQArABIIACAw%3D%3D#amp_tf=From%20%251%24s&aoh=16553032818209&referrer=https%3A%2F%2Fwww.google.com&share=https%3A%2F%2Fwww.medindia.net%2Fpatients%2Flifestyleandwellness%2Fjuices-for-detoxification-and-wellbeing-disease-prevention-and-cure.htm

Levko, R. (2021, December 1). *Juicing and Pregnancy: Is Juicing Safe For Pregnant Women?* Tastylicious. Retrieved June 28, 2022, from https://tastylicious.com/juicing-and-pregnancy-is-juicing-safe-for-pregnant-women/

Schaefer, A. (2018, December 4). *Juicing vs. Blending: Which Is Better for Me?* Healthline. Retrieved June 28, 2022, from https://www.healthline.com/health/food-nutrition/juicing-vs-blending#:%7E:text=The%20difference%20between%20juicing%20and%20blending%20is%20what's%20left%20out,that%20bulks%20up%20the%20product .

Printed in the USA
CPSIA information can be obtained
at www.ICGtesting.com
LVHW080052130823
754935LV00012B/331